"*Golden Rules for Vibrant Health* is a treasure. Between its covers is the wisdom of a gifted doctor's lifetime. Dr. Sweere offers a remarkably comprehensive, well-grounded set of health recommendations, along with something even more precious—a model of a doctor who truly listens, growing as he learns from his patients. Those who read his book will gain valuable health information along with a deepened understanding of what truly matters in life."

—DANIEL REDWOOD, D.C., AUTHOR, *A TIME TO HEAL* AND *FUNDAMENTALS OF CHIROPRACTIC*

"*Golden Rules for Vibrant Health* is a valuable educational resource for the general public offering a broad array of wellness measures. Dr. Sweere is an experienced educator and wellness advocate. Any person could greatly benefit from reading this book, applying the information and concepts contained therein. As Dr. Sweere points out, if you don't take the time and effort to be well, you will have to take the time to be sick. I highly recommend this book to any doctor to read for themselves and as a resource for their patients. Application of its principles will minimize the need for medications and crisis oriented medical care."

—NORMAN M. HORNS, M.D., ASSOCIATE PROFESSOR, CLINICAL AND BASIC SCIENCES
NORTHWESTERN HEALTH SCIENCES UNIVERSITY

"In this time of ever-increasing healthcare costs, both companies as well as individuals are faced with difficult decisions on how to better manage their health and wellness. Dr. Sweere's *Golden Rules for Vibrant Health* provides the needed information and impetus for all who care about their health. Those who are willing to apply the principles outlined in his book will find the time and money well worth the investment."

—STEPHEN R. LARSON, PRESIDENT, LARSON CONSULTING, INC.

"*Golden Rules for Vibrant Health* is a book of lifestyle guidelines for those who want to improve their health and avoid illnesses that necessitate dependence on drugs. The public needs sound, accurate advice that they can trust to guide them in their healthy lifestyle decisions. This book is the best set of guidelines and advice available."

—DANIEL J. MURPHY, D.C., CLINICAL SCIENCES FACULTY, LIFE CHIROPRACTIC COLLEGE WEST

"No Golden Rule is more important tha
This is a book to help you truly love yourself as wel

T0273478

—C. NORMAN SHEALY, M.D., PH.D., FOUNDING PRESIDENT, AMERICA
PRESIDENT, HOLOS INSTITUTES OF HEALTH, INC. • PRESIDENT, HOLOS UNIVERSITY GRADUATE SEMINARY

"This book is yet another accomplishment in Dr. Sweere's very successful lifetime. He lives by his word, and now he shares those words of wisdom with us in this book. It summarizes ideas and philosophies known to improve the health and well-being of the whole person. Dr. Sweere's influence has made a positive difference in my life as well as the lives of my patients. I highly recommend this book to any person desiring a healthier, happier life."

—JOHN D. LAUGHLIN III, D.D.S., PAST PRESIDENT,
AMERICAN HOLISTIC DENTAL ASSOCIATION

"Dr. Sweere's book is the most comprehensive holistic guidebook I've seen. Most health-related books focus on just physiological topics, or just psycho-spiritual matters, but his covers the whole spectrum of life. The information is very practical and down-to-earth, giving readers specific actions he or she can follow to become healthier. I highly recommend it."

—CHERYL HAWK, D.C., PH.D., PROFESSOR

"Practical. Simple. Profound. With brilliant simplicity, *Golden Rules for Vibrant Health* weaves a broad scope of healing modalities and resources into a practical and usable manual for creating a life of increased quality and richness. Truly unique in embracing all facets of health—including body, mind, and sprit, this book provides the reader with a wealth of information in an elegantly simple and clear format. As a health and wellness educator, I highly recommend this book as a powerful tool to provide clients a wholistic and comprehensive source of practical health guidelines and the inspiration to make the daily choices that create a healthy and fulfilling life. This book is a must-have for any practitioner to empower their clients to take an active role in their health and well-being."

—CHRISTY MOLITOR, D.C., COMMUNITY AND CORPORATE HEALTH AND WELLNESS EDUCATOR

"I am tremendously impressed, but not surprised with the breadth, depth, and credibility of the healthful living information and guidance Dr. Sweere's book provides. If I were still in private practice, I would make special efforts to make my patients aware of this book and the positive direction it would give for their everyday living. It holds much promise for being able to transform lives."

—JOHN F. ALLENBURG, D.C., PRESIDENT EMERITUS,
NORTHWESTERN HEALTH SCIENCES UNIVERSITY

GOLDEN RULES FOR VIBRANT HEALTH IN BODY, MIND, AND *SPIRIT*

A HOLISTIC APPROACH TO HEALTH AND WELLNESS

JOSEPH J. SWEERE, D.C.

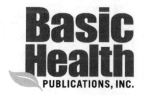

Basic Health PUBLICATIONS, INC.

The information contained in this book is based upon the research and personal and professional experiences of the author. It is not intended as a substitute for consulting with your physician or other healthcare provider. Any attempt to diagnose and treat an illness should be done under the direction of a healthcare professional.

The publisher does not advocate the use of any particular healthcare protocol but believes the information in this book should be available to the public. The publisher and author are not responsible for any adverse effects or consequences resulting from the use of the suggestions, preparations, or procedures discussed in this book. Should the reader have any questions concerning the appropriateness of any procedures or preparation mentioned, the author and the publisher strongly suggest consulting a professional healthcare advisor.

Basic Health Publications, Inc.
28812 Top of the World Drive
Laguna Beach, CA 92651
949-715-7327

Library of Congress Cataloging-in-Publication Data

Sweere, Joseph J.
  Golden rules for vibrant health in body, mind, and spirit : a holistic approach to health and wellness / Joseph J. Sweere.
      p. cm.
  Includes bibliographical references and index.
  ISBN-13: 9781-59120-077-2
  ISBN-10: 1-59120-077-6
 1. Health. 2. Holistic medicine. 3. Self-care, Health. I. Title.

  R733.S98   2004
  613—dc22

                              2004007271

Editor: Roberta W. Waddell
Typesetting/Book design: Gary A. Rosenberg
Cover design: Mike Stromberg

Printed in the United States of America

10   9   8   7   6   5   4   3

Contents

Acknowledgments, xi

Foreword, xiii

The Golden Rule, xvii

Introduction, 1

1. Food: What and How You Eat, 3

2. Water and Your Body, 11

3. Structure and Function: Exercising and Maintaining
   Your Body, 17

4. Alkalinity and Acidity: The Right Ratio for
   Your Body, 25

5. Medicinal Wonder Foods, 31

6. Nutritional Supplements, 37

7. Rest and Sleep, 45

8. Fresh Air and Breathing, 55

9. Choosing Your Doctors and Care Providers, 61

10. Don't Put Poisons into Your Body, 81

11. Heart Disease and Stroke, 95

12. Blood Sugar Disorders, 103

13. Headaches, 111

14. Managing Your Weight, 119

15. Arthritis, 125

16. Cancer—A Modern Plague, 133

17. Constipation, 141

18. Asthma and Respiratory Disorders, 145

19. Depression, 149

20. Colds, Flu, and Other Infections, 155

21. Stress Management, 161

22. Relationships, 173

23. Common Sense, 185

24. Ergonomics, 199

25. Your Attitudes and Belief Systems, 207

Notable Quotes—Wise Instructions for Life, 221

Conclusion, 223

References, 225

Recommended Reading, 231

Resources and Websites, 233

Index, 239

About the Author, 253

When health is absent,
wisdom cannot reveal itself,
art cannot become manifest,
strength cannot be exerted,
wealth becomes useless,
and reason is powerless.

—HEROPHILUS, 300 B.C.

Dedication

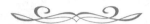

This work is dedicated to my family. The extraordinary love, patience, support, and encouragement that come from a caring and sharing family are without equal. Special acknowledgment is extended to my late parents, Cornelius and Gertrude, who lived, practiced, and inspired most of the commonsense principles expressed in this book. Also, my brothers, Ted, Harry, Ed, and David, and my sister, Veronica, who shared in our parents' ancestral legacy. And, especially my wife, Mary, and our children, Michael, Melissa, Steven, Craig, Jonathan, and Ryan, and their children, Mitchell, Michael, Alison, Eliot, and Benjamin, who are the products of our sacred covenant. Thank you for the joy you have brought into my life.

Acknowledgments

eartfelt gratitude is extended to the many people who helped make this book become a reality. Some have served in extraordinary ways, and special ongoing thanks is extended to Elizabeth Auppl, Monica Auppl, Naomi Goodwin, Marilee Pfarr, Mary Beth Martin, Drs. Barry Bradley, Robert Bruley, Lyle Coleman, Steve Dandrea, Linda Dobberstein, Robert Dubro, and Mary Forte. Also, Doctors David Geary, Stephanie Geary, Betsy Lavin, Norman Horns, John Laughlin, Jeffrey Rich, Michael Schurch, Mary Tuchscherer, Richard Vincent, and Sharon Williams, as well as Registered Nurses Deborah Miller, Kris Pirkl, Romana Wesely, and Lucy Coleman. All of these people provided invaluable constructive feedback and editing suggestions for which I am most appreciative.

Other professional colleagues deserve applause for reviewing various sections and early drafts of the manuscript, including Doctors William Elkington, Chad Henriksen, Rob Krege, Link Larson, Ed Mauer, Mark Leutem, Gary Miller, Michael Peterson, and Nevin Rosenberg.

For helpful feedback regarding the perspectives of consumers, students, and other readers who may not have a scientific background, my thanks go to Cynthia Bellini-Olsen, Jac Daccardi, Chris Davis, Jueli Gastworth, Brian and Catherine Halliday, Jack Hockenberry, Steve Larson, Carrie Oleston, Jerry and Sharon Peterson, Brenda Schuler, Breck Stovern, Barbara Thompson, Sara M. (Moe) Smith, and Winona Watkins.

Gracious acknowledgment is also extended to the administration, faculty, students, and staff of Northwestern Health Sciences University. Thank you for the patience and understanding you have provided during the hundreds of hours of preparation required for development of this work. No words can fully describe my gratitude.

Great admiration, respect, and gratitude is due to all those pioneering healthcare practitioners, regardless of their professional discipline, who have dedicated their lives to advancing the cause of natural, holistic approaches to healing throughout the ages. Surely the world will greatly benefit from your collective courage, dedication, and perseverance, often provided unselfishly, in spite of significant criticism and even professional ostracism from the popular orthodoxy of the time. May your God richly reward each and every one of you.

In addition, I wish to express gratitude to the thousands of patients I have had the privilege of serving throughout the years. Thank you for the confidence you have shown in my care and the many gestures of kindness you have bestowed upon me. Your health crises have been my greatest motivation for the creation of this book, and your recoveries, large and small, have served as my greatest inspiration.

Finally, I wish to acknowledge profound appreciation to Bobby Waddell, Editor, and Norman Goldfind, Publisher of Basic Health Publications. It is thanks to each of them that this book has become a reality. The support, patience, guidance, and assistance they have provided are deeply appreciated. So, Norm and Bobby, please accept my special thanks and know that I will always have a warm space in my heart for your kindness. I have greatly enjoyed working with you.

To all who have helped, and also to those whom I may have inadvertently overlooked, I extend my deep and sincere thanks, with my best wishes for a long, healthy, and happy life.

Foreword

For nearly three decades, it has been my privilege to know Dr. Joseph Sweere, both professionally and as a dear friend to me and my family. Having been afforded many ongoing opportunities to work with Dr. Sweere on common-interest projects over the years, I am honored to provide the foreword comments prior to your reading what he shares on these pages.

This book is about preventing disruptions to experiencing life at its fullest, by embracing that which is healthful, prudent, and naturally kind to the human body, mind, spirit, and soul. The words throughout this book reflect the unpretentious, vibrant, and energetic nature of the author.

Dr. Sweere is the embodiment of life, love, peace, and joy. His life is an inspiration for so many people, and an example of abundant living by practicing wisdom in making life choices. His passion for life is exceeded only by his compassion for humankind and his ability to live the golden rule. He practices what he preaches, and now you, too, can embark on a path to make your life the best it can be for yourself and your loved ones. Perhaps you have heard the cliché that, sometimes, the books we read choose us. By this token, since you have picked up this book, I know that you are also a health-conscious person in the daily pursuit of the highest-quality life possible.

You will find that following the practices recommended in these pages will help you absorb the golden rules into your whole being and allow you to continue to be your very best you for the world and your loved ones.

—Elizabeth L. Auppl

Hands with a Heart
A HOLISTIC HEALTHCARE CENTER

Invites You to Attend
a Two-Hour Health and
Wellness Conference

❋ Learn the Golden Rules
for Healthful Living

❋ Health Questions Answered

❋ Bring a Friend

TUESDAY EVENING • 7–9 P.M.
COMMUNITY EDUCATION CENTER

Think of this book as your invitation to attend the type of health and wellness educational forum described above. If you find this book of value, please feel welcome to share the information contained within. For many it could be lifesaving.

The Golden Rule

DO UNTO OTHERS AS YOU WOULD HAVE THEM DO UNTO YOU.

"Doing unto others" is fun, easy, and wonderfully rewarding. In fact, it is the means through which we enjoy almost everything that we cherish as valuable and meaningful in our lives. Doing unto others is fun and easy, as long as you are healthy and able.

When you are sick, or not feeling well, most of your thoughts tend to turn inward and you may become self-oriented. Often, when an illness is not relieved in a couple of days or even weeks, it becomes chronic and progressively more debilitating, perhaps causing the sick person to become dependent upon others. Sickness and disease make us less and less able to enjoy life's abundance, or to fulfill our maximum potential.

The greatest gift you can give others is your best you—your *healthiest* you. The greatest gift a husband and wife can give each other is optimal health. The greatest gift parents can give their children is vibrant health in body, mind, and spirit. This is true for everyone: workers to employers, employers to workers; coaches to athletes, athletes to coaches; teachers to students, students to teachers; and so on, regardless of who you are or what you do. Optimal health is also the greatest gift you can give *yourself.* Therefore, consider adding the following concept to the Golden Rule: "Do unto *yourself* as you would have others do unto you."

The Golden Rules for Vibrant Health in Body, Mind, and Spirit was written for health-conscious people who wish to reach their maximum human potential. It was also written for people who are currently not enjoying optimal health and wish to overcome illness in order to restore energy, vitality, and well-being. Consider that a candle's light and warmth burns as brightly on its last day as on its first. It doesn't flicker and sputter when it still has half its wax. My goal is to provide you with practical information and tools that will allow you to enjoy life completely and fully from the first day to the last.

Optimum health is a manifestation of harmony of body, mind, and spirit.

y hope is that the guidelines presented in *The Golden Rules for Vibrant Health in Body, Mind, and Spirit* will have significant value regardless of your age, gender, or station in life—young or old, male or female, rich or poor. As you reflect on the information and suggestions in each chapter, you will likely come to realize that it's not so much how old you are, or how wealthy you are, but how *well* you are that largely determines your happiness. A common regret among people as they grow older is the wish that they had taken better care of themselves when they were younger. It is encouraging to note, however, that it is *never too late* to begin your journey toward improved health and better quality of life. Even small steps along this path—such as avoiding caffeine, drinking more pure water, and going for walks—can help you achieve remarkable changes. You will feel great pride in the positive changes you make and will find them progressively more enjoyable as you experience more vibrant health.

In the year 1900, about one person out of every fifty developed cancer. Today, one out of every *three* will be diagnosed with this killer disease. And a host of other conditions—Alzheimer's disease, asthma, birth defects, diabetes digestive disorders, infertility, miscarriages, multiple sclerosis, Parkinson's disease, and vascular disorders, to name a few—are increasing in incidence and severity despite the vast amounts of money, time, talent, and resources devoted to human health. The economic effect this has on our society is enormous, and the associated cost in pain and suffering can't even be measured. It's estimated that one trillion, six-hundred billion dollars was spent on health care in the United States in 2003. Broken down, the per capita expenditure ($3,724 for every man, woman, and child) greatly exceeds that of any other country, and yet, among developed countries, the health status of Americans ranks thirty-seventh, according to the World Health Organization (WHO).

Introduction

Most everyone can appreciate the security and peace of mind that comes with having sufficient health and life insurance policies. Similarly, the golden rules may be considered a form of health or life insurance. Although the insurance company will pay a portion of your expenses when you need crisis-related medical care or injury management and will also pay a death benefit if you die, sending a check to an insurance company for your health or life insurance does absolutely nothing to assure your health or your life because neither form of insurance will help protect your health or prevent you from becoming ill, injured, or experiencing an untimely death. But barring involvement in a natural disaster or catastrophic accident, your dedicated application of the principles in this book will give you a better chance for optimal health and a long, enjoyable life. As you begin to explore and absorb this information, you may experience an overriding feeling of, "What if I can't or don't follow all these rules?" Let me put your mind at ease. I suggest that you think of these recommendations as guidelines rather than strict rules that are never to be broken. Even though the value of these rules may be golden, they are not meant to be commandments. Becoming stressed about an occasional inappropriate choice you may make is more apt to harm your health than the indiscretion itself. To the degree you can, simply follow the rules and trust in your body's powerful innate wisdom, and its ability to protect and heal itself. By doing so, you will have earned the privilege of fully enjoying life and living to your unique maximum potential. This is my goal and my desire for you. Best wishes!

GOLDEN RULES FOR ATTAINING AND MAINTAINING VIBRANT HEALTH AND VITALITY

The body you are given will be yours for the duration of your time here.
Love it or hate it, accept it or reject it, it is the only one you will receive in this lifetime.
It will be with you from the moment you draw your first breath, to the last beat of
your heart. Since there is a no refund, no exchange policy on this body of yours,
it is essential that you learn to transform your body from a mere vessel into a
beloved partner and lifelong ally, as the relationship between you and your
body is the most fundamental and important relationship of your lifetime.
It is the blue-print from which all your other relationships will be built.

—CHERIE CARTER-SCOTT, *IF LIFE IS A GAME, THESE ARE THE RULES*

1. Food:
What and How You Eat

his first Golden Rule of good health that we will discuss pertains to your relationship with food as a primary source of energy and health. From ancient times, human survival on the earth has depended almost exclusively on the availability of adequate food sources. The human body has the ability to obtain nourishment from a very wide range of plants and animals. Agribusiness, which includes the cultivation and harvesting of plants and animals for human food consumption is currently the single largest industry in the world. In your desire to maintain optimal health, the importance of food, including how it is produced, transported, processed, preserved, stored, selected, and prepared, cannot be overemphasized.

The following suggestions will be helpful in optimizing the conversion of the foods you eat into the energy you need to sustain your life and preserve your health and well-being.

EATING MEALS

Chew Your Food

Digestion begins in your mouth and proper digestion of food is very important for maintaining health and energy. Chew your food thoroughly, and eat slowly. A simple rule to follow is to completely chew and swallow what you have already put in your mouth before taking another bite. From time to time as you are eating, put your fork or spoon down on the table as a reminder of this.

Don't Wash It Down

Drinking large amounts of beverages with your meals dilutes the chemistry of your saliva, as well as the fluids in your stomach and gastrointestinal tract that are needed for the proper digestion, absorption, and assimilation of foods. Avoid drinking large quantities of water, milk, coffee, sodas, or other liquids one-half hour before and two hours after eating.

Give Thanks

In addition to thanking your creator, be grateful to the food that is sacrificing its life so you can live. Silently say, "Thank you, carrot," "Thank you, fish," "Thank you, cow." And while you are at it, also say, "Thank you, farmer" or "Thank you, fisherman."

Enjoy Your Meals

Sit down while you eat. Turn off the TV. Whether at a simple meal or a banquet, eat with great pleasure and great gratitude. Enjoy the company at your table, and if you eat alone, enjoy your solitude.

Assist Your Digestion

It is not a good idea to eat when you are angry and upset, or when you are very tired. Digestion is best accomplished in a peaceful, relaxed, hearts-filled-with-gratitude environment. Proper digestion ensures an adequate supply of nutrients needed by your trillions of body cells to perform their important work in maintaining your health.

Avoid Chewing Gum

The mechanical action of chewing stimulates the production of saliva, which contains specific chemicals manufactured by the glands and cells in the mouth to aid in the digestion of sugars, starches, and other carbohydrate foods. While most chewing gum contains sugar, it is not meant to be swallowed and digested. As you chew gum, however, the saliva that your glands secrete for digestion is continuously swallowed, along with the sugar. This mix enters your stomach and alters and dilutes the delicately balanced chemistry of the stomach and upper-digestive-tract juices. This can, in turn, disturb the proper digestion of proteins, such as beans, cheese, eggs, fish, meats, and so forth.

In addition, people who chew gum almost always have a dominant chewing side. Thus, if you often chew gum, you may be using one side of your jaw and chewing muscles much more than the other—without even realizing it. This overuse can result in fatigue, stress, and eventually an uneven wear pattern of your teeth and jaw musculature that can lead to problems in your temporo-mandibular joint (TMJ). The symptoms of TMJ can be both painful and annoying, and may include headaches and ear, nose, throat, and sinus disorders.

Just Say, "No Thank You"

In spite of all the poverty and hunger in our world today, more people die of diseases related to overweight and obesity than of starvation. In fact, second only to Bible sales, the two most popular types of books sold in America today are cookbooks and diet or weight-loss books. Therefore, I can't stress enough how important it is to eat only when you are hungry and eat in moderation, without overstuffing yourself. When offered a second helping, or a gooey dessert, just say, "No, thank you."

HAVE RESPECT FOR NATURE'S DESIGN

From time to time, particularly during mealtime, it is good to reflect on the grandeur of your existence. Consider that, within nature's awesome mysteries and complexities, the secrets of life and health are really very simple. Life originates exclusively from four sources: the food you eat, the air you breathe, the water you drink, and the sun that warms you. This is true for you, and for almost every life form on earth. Tree, snail, polar bear, honeybee—all depend on this simple formula, and paying attention to it can help ensure a long, healthy, vibrant, and productive life.

OVERFED AND UNDERNOURISHED

Most Americans are overfed with calorie-rich, nutrient-poor, fatty, starchy, sweetened, prepackaged, overprocessed, and artificially preserved junk foods. And while an almost epidemic obesity is the result of this type of diet, most overweight people are still *undernourished* at the cellular level. Cellular starvation results in continuous craving for what is lacking and creates a vicious cycle of overeating, weight gain, fad diets, and potentially dangerous weight-loss experimentation.

Most cravings can be overcome by providing the body with the nutrients it needs. Obtaining and consuming the proper balance of nutrients is perhaps the most significant contribution a person can make to maintaining vibrant health and optimal energy, and preventing disease. Does this seem like common sense to you? For many, this idea can be somewhat confusing and challenging. How can the average American, essentially untrained in nutrition, decide on an optimal nutritional program for good health? It's not always easy to know what's best for your individual needs, particularly if you have special nutritional concerns—for example, if you are pregnant or have diabetes or food allergies. An example of this is the role of a readily available B vitamin, folic acid (folate), in the prevention of the birth-defect disease known as spina bifida. Up to 75 percent of all severe cases of this condition can be *prevented* simply by providing women of childbearing age with adequate amounts of folic acid before and during pregnancy. Although this is a practical and inexpensive thing to do, the majority of the public lacks the level of nutritional awareness to do it.

So how do you ensure that you're getting the proper balance of nutrients for optimal health? I recommend you carefully choose a personal nutritional consultant, just as you would your personal physician. You may wish to visit a holistically trained healthcare provider who is well-versed in clinical nutrition. If you have special needs beyond his or her expertise, ask your doctor to refer you to an expert nutritional consultant in your community.

My personal nutritional consultant is my friend and colleague Dr. Barry Bradley, a chiropractic physician who also holds a Ph.D. in clinical nutrition. His book *10 Hidden Reasons You Are Sick—and What to Do about Them* is an excellent reference for all who want to enjoy better health through balanced nutrition.

CHOOSE YOUR FOODS WISELY
Organic Foods

Whole, fresh, natural foods are more healthful than artificially preserved, commercially packaged, processed, refined, radiated, and genetically engineered foods grown in soils contaminated by artificial fertilizers, herbicides, and insecticides. Therefore, I recommend that you purchase a wide variety of organically grown foods. To be sure that you're getting what you pay for, look for foods that are labeled "USDA Organic." The words "all natural" mean very little in this regard. According to the United States Department of Agriculture (USDA), the 100 percent organic label may be used on products that contain 100 percent organically produced ingredients. Products sold simply as "organic" must contain at least 95 percent organically produced ingredients. Foods that are sold with the label "made with organic ingredients" must contain at least 70 percent organic ingredients.

Eating a diet that includes a variety of well-balanced, organically grown whole foods is an excellent way to ensure the generous supply of natural vitamins, minerals, enzymes, fiber, herbs, and oils that your body needs for optimal health. As most organic farmers do, I believe that "grass fed is best." Many foods, especially those known to have a high protein content—dairy, beef, pork, and poultry—should be derived from animals and birds raised in surroundings as close as possible to their natural environment, such as open air pastures and grasslands. Unfortunately, particularly in the United States, many such foods are obtained from livestock raised in very crowded, factory-style settings. These animals are continuously fed antibiotics to prevent contagious diseases, feed additives that contain hormones, and other substances designed to accelerate growth and make them more profitable. These chemicals ultimately become part of the human food chain and add stress to all the body's systems, negatively affecting health and longevity. It's not surprising that such unnatural farm practices are considered to be so controversial. In addition to the health risks of consuming such foods, commercial farm practices that keep large numbers of livestock confined in cramped quarters result in significant and potentially toxic waste runoff, and add greatly to the contamination of the earth's soil and our drinking water supply.

Wash Your Produce and Peel Your Fruits

When organically grown produce is not available, it is a good practice to carefully wash your vegetables and peel your fruits, although it may not always be possible to remove all residues of fungicides, herbicides, pesticides, and waxes. Environne Fruit and Vegetable Wash is an excellent product available in health food stores and the natural foods section of your supermarket that can be a great help in removing most traces of residue.

Avoid Irradiated Foods

As much as possible, I recommend you refrain from purchasing and eating foods that have been exposed to radiation in order to destroy various strains of potentially harmful microorganisms, such as E. coli. Since irradiated foods do not spoil as readily and therefore have a longer shelf life than foods that are not processed in this way, you can understand why food manufacturers and processors often promote food irradiation. But irradiated foods potentially have health risks, particularly to susceptible individuals and perhaps to our future offspring. Since the long-range health effects of irradiation are as yet unknown, it is best to choose foods that have not been irradiated whenever you can.

Avoid Genetically Engineered Foods

Genetic engineering is the practice of intentionally altering or manipulating the essential blueprints of living species, including those of plants, animals, and microorganisms. Using this technology largely for profit, bioengineering companies develop and then patent such products and sell them on the open market, promising that the technology can eliminate world hunger, cure diseases, and make virtually all crops resistant to pests and weeds, and therefore inestimably superior and highly valuable for improved public health. What most of the public doesn't realize, however, is that this revolutionary new gene-splicing technology is still in its very early stages of development, and virtually nothing is known about the potential long-term health and environmental dangers of genetically modified foods. A number of common foods and plant-related products are already on the market, with many more in various stages of development.

Among the most controversial of the current food technologies is bovine growth hormone (BGH), which is injected into dairy cows to stimulate them to produce more milk. Because of the raging debate among scientists, and a growing concern about links to increased risks of cancer and other diseases, both Canada and the European Union have banned the use of BGH.

Currently, more than four dozen genetically engineered foods and crops are being grown or sold in the United States, including canola oil, corn, cottonseed oil, dairy products, papaya, potatoes, squash, and tomatoes. While many highly respected scientists have expressed grave concerns about the potential threat to human and plant health, these products do not require special labeling and can therefore be routinely purchased by uninformed consumers in regular food stores and supermarkets.

You may be aware of the deadly viruses and bacteria that have formed mutant strains capable of resisting even the most potent forms of antibiotics and antiviral medicines. These appropriately named "superbug microorganisms" actually developed in response to man's attempts to eradicate them. As all other living species on the earth, microorganisms have an inborn need to survive. When threatened by external forces such as the overuse of germ-killing anti- biotics, it triggered the microbe's survival mechanism in such a way that it re- sulted in the creation of mutations of the organisms whose offspring then became immune or resistant to such threats. These highly virulent strains of mutant microbes now pose a significant threat to the human immune system. Because of this, there is genuine concern on the part of world health authorities that humankind may once again be teetering on the brink of non-stoppable plagues similar to those that destroyed many millions of people in the past. Using the same reasoning, many scientists are concerned that the dream of genetically altering the DNA of plant crop seeds for the purpose of making them immune to harmful insect and weed infestation may backfire. It is feared that similar to what has happened as the result of man's war against germs, mutant strains of highly dangerous, noxious pests and weed plants will crop up, thus greatly com- pounding the original problem.

Notable health risks associated with genetically engineered foods have been documented in a variety of respected scientific studies and reports. Worldwide

controversy continues to grow regarding the environmental, health, and socioe-
conomic risks of human bioengineering of food and food-related products. For
these reasons, it is my belief that you can best protect your health by avoiding
genetically engineered foods. Because labeling of genetically engineered foods
is not yet required, the only reasonable way to do this is to boycott such products altogether by *purchasing certified organic food products whenever possible*.
To learn more about the controversy surrounding genetically engineered food
and food-related products, do a search for "Genetically Engineered Foods" on
the Internet.

THE VEGETARIAN DIET

People who follow vegetarian diets restrict their consumption of animal flesh,
including fish and fowl, in any form. Vegans also restrict their consumption of
animal products, such as butter, cheese, eggs, and milk. Sometimes the vegetarian way of life is motivated by spiritual objectives, but vegetarians often make
these life changes for their health and well-being. No matter what the reason,
however, there is some debate regarding the health outcomes of the vegetarian
or vegan disciplines.

A primary issue for the vegetarian is the risk of deficiency in a variety of critical nutrients required by the body for vibrant health and vitality. Because strict
vegetarians avoid all animal products, they run a very significant risk of developing protein deficiency, as well as deficiencies of the B vitamins, and iron and
other minerals. Protein is a major component of every cell in the body, including those of the blood, bones, hair, muscles, nails, nerves, skin, and all of these
internal organs. Additionally, protein is absolutely critical for the production of
enzymes and hormones the body needs for regulation and reproduction.

Protein is available from vegetables, fruits, and other nonanimal sources
including nuts, seeds, whole grains, and beans, and soy and its soy products.
Unfortunately, almost none of these food sources, even in combination, provide
a complete balance of all the amino acids, vitamins, minerals, enzymes, and
other nutrients required by the body for optimal health. Therefore, if you decide
to continue a vegetarian lifestyle after weighing all the facts, you will need to
understand your nutritional needs and take extra steps to make sure you're taking in a healthy balance of essential nutrients. For example, you may need
to supplement your protein intake with high-protein vegetable foods, such as
spirulina and others. In addition, if you wish to maintain a strictly vegetarian
lifestyle, you may need to undergo periodic laboratory tests to monitor your
nutritional health status.

Best Sources of Non-Vegetable Protein

A balanced daily ration of any of the following high-protein food sources listed below is recommended:

- Dairy products
- Eggs
- Fish
- Lamb (from healthy young lambs)
- *Lean* red meat (from young, healthy, free-range, grass-fed beef cattle)
- Range-fed (free-range) chicken and turkey
- Seafoods

Lean red beef contains more amino acids, B vitamins, iron, zinc, and other needed minerals in the correct ratio for the body's needs than any other known food. As we already discussed, when available, certified organic sources are best.

FOODS ARE YOUR BEST MEDICINE

Hippocrates, the Father of Medicine, said, "Let your foods be your medicines; and let your medicines be your foods." A 1997 USDA survey titled *How Americans Spend Their Food Dollars* found that the ten items generating the highest sales, or most money spent, in grocery stores in America were as follows:

1. Marlboro cigarettes
2. Coca Cola Classic
3. Kraft Macaroni and Cheese
4. Pepsi Cola
5. Diet Coke
6. Budweiser beer
7. Campbell's soup
8. Tide detergent
9. Folger's coffee
10. Winston cigarettes

How does your grocery list compare?

2. Water and Your Body

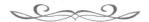

Although the average human being can live up to three weeks without food, a person can only live about three days without water. It is absolutely the most essential nutrient for life and our very existence on earth. The next Golden Rule of good health concerns your relationship with water.

STAYING HYDRATED

Most Americans are dehydrated, largely due to the diuretics contained in many of the popular drinks we consume. A *diuretic* is any chemical that stimulates the loss of fluids from the body. Caffeine and alcohol are good examples of these substances. Many Americans wake up in the morning and need their coffee—one, two, or even three cups is common even before we're out the door. At work, perhaps another cup of coffee, or a caffeinated soft drink, which also has a diuretic effect. Lunch? More coffee or soft drinks and more of the same in the mid-afternoon hours. At dinner, we may relax with a glass or two of wine, or some other dehydrating alcoholic drink. This very common practice has a continuous diuretic, dehydrating effect on all the body's cells.

Staying hydrated is really very easy. All you need to do is drink lots of pure, fresh, mineral-rich water every single day. A simple way to do this is to make it a daily practice to consume one-half of your body weight in ounces of water. For example, if you weigh 160 pounds, you should drink 80 ounces—or ten 8-ounce glasses of water daily. You will need to drink more water if you are athletic, your work is physically demanding, or you work or play in an unusually warm or hot environment. But even if you work in an office, your body may lose approximately ten glasses, 80 ounces, of water each day through perspiration, respiration, and urination. All of this must be replenished to avoid dehydration.

Water as a Body Cleanser

Water is the primary means by which the body cleanses itself, internally and externally. Obviously, when you take a bath or shower to cleanse the outside of your body, you prefer to use clean, fresh water. The same logic would hold true for cleansing, or detoxifying, the cells on the inside of your body. Can you picture taking a refreshing, cleansing shower with strong black coffee or perhaps tasty, sugary soda? In essence, this is the bath you are giving all the cells and vital organs of your body when these products are the only liquids you ingest. To the extent possible, try to avoid products that contain caffeine, such as coffee, caffeinated teas, and chocolate. This also holds true for most soft drinks because, in addition to a host of artificial colorings, a variety of unhealthy acids, and sugar or artificial sweeteners, many of these beverages are laced with caffeine. Alcohol is also a diuretic and so when you drink beer, wine, or mixed drinks, these beverages can actually cause your body to lose more fluids than you are taking in.

Bathing vs. Showering

Is there any health advantage to taking a shower rather than a bath? Many people enjoy long soaks in a tub of hot, soapy water, which can be very relaxing and can certainly have therapeutic benefits, especially if a whirlpool effect is generated. However, when you soak in a hot tub for any length of time, your body sheds billions of dead skin cells and bacteria, as well as dirt, perspiration, and other impurities and toxins discharged from the body via the skin. Given this, I believe that showering is healthier and more effective than taking a bath. Your reward will be cleaner, healthier skin and fewer urinary tract infections. However, if you do decide to enjoy a nice, hot bath every now and again, keep in mind that it's a good idea to rinse yourself thoroughly in the shower after your bath.

Water for Spine and Joint Health

The discs of the spine are water-filled, hydraulic-like devices that require appropriate hydration for their efficient shock-absorbing and load-bearing function. All the tendons and joints of the body are lubricated by synovial fluid, a slippery substance composed mainly of water. In light of this, you can understand how disc degeneration and herniation, joint disorders, muscle aches and pains, and tendonitis can be aggravated by—if not caused by—drinking too little water. In fact, many ill health and disease conditions can result from inadequate water intake. For more on the importance of water to spine and joint health, I recommend reading *Your Body's Many Cries for Water* by Dr. F. Batmanghelidj.

Water and Aging

Want to avoid wrinkles? Make sure your body is well hydrated. Consider a fresh, ripe plum, and then consider a prune. Consider a juicy grape, and then a raisin. The only difference is hydration. Wrinkles are an expression of the skin's internal cell structure, and the skin reflects the condition throughout the body.

Since water constitutes about 70 percent of the body, a constant, readily available supply of water is required for every single one of its several trillion cells to efficiently transport nutrients and eliminate wastes for optimal health and maximum longevity. Have you noticed that, as people grow older, they become shorter and gradually lose their body mass? One of the consequences of a lifetime of dehydration is shrinking tissue cells and the gradual breakdown and deterioration of the body's tissues.

Water and Your Jangled Nerves

Want to keep your cool, stay more relaxed, and sleep better? Drink more pure water. People who drink a lot of coffee and soft drinks come home from work buzzed up from the caffeine and sugar, and they want to relax. Often their solution is to reach into the refrigerator or liquor cabinet for a drink containing alcohol. However, as you already learned, alcohol actually promotes tissue dehydration and an additional buildup of toxic wastes in the body. People who do not rely on alcohol to relax may remain wound up from their caffeine and sugar intake during the day, making sleep at night difficult. Resorting to sleeping pills only results in a drug-induced, restless sleep and, upon waking, a perceived need for more caffeine, kicking off another sugar-caffeine, up-down, roller-coaster day.

Water Substitutes

In addition to pure water and fresh fruit and vegetable juices, there are other healthy beverages you can drink, such as skim milk and caffeine-free herbal teas. If you enjoy fruit juices, freshly squeezed and organically grown are best. However, when this is not an option for you, be sure to choose all-natural, 100 percent pure fruit juices or juice concentrates. Be aware that frozen juice concentrates are higher in vitamin C than canned or bottled pasteurized juices. Some experts maintain that the acids in fruit juices react chemically and have a leaching effect when bottled and stored in plastic, aluminum, or other metal-alloy containers, so juices in glass containers or waxed-paper cartons are probably safer.

With very few exceptions, fruits and fruit juices have an alkalizing effect on your body chemistry at the cellular level, which is highly desirable. This includes citrus fruits and juices—oranges, lemons, limes, and grapefruit. By choosing a wide variety of fruits and fruit juices, you are giving your body the opportunity to select the nutrients it requires for good health and optimal energy. Trust its wisdom to do so.

Other Popular Beverages: Decaf Coffee, Soft Drinks, and Diet Sodas

Did you know that a twelve-ounce can of Classic Coca-Cola contains *eleven* teaspoons of sugar? Drinking three cans a day of the "Real Thing," the world's most popular soft drink, is equivalent to eating thirty-three teaspoons of sugar, a good-sized bowlful. However, as harmful as consuming too much sugar can be, you should also avoid diet sodas and artificial sweeteners of all kinds, as well as foods that contain artificial sweeteners, as these substances have been associated with a variety of neurological disorders, including seizures, and the symptoms of multiple sclerosis. Other detrimental health risks associated with artificial sweeteners include allergic reactions, headaches, nervousness, and yeast infections.

A Harvard University study in the June 2000 *Archives of Pediatrics and Adolescent Medicine* suggests that carbonated beverages, especially colas, may weaken bone structure. Among 460 ninth- and tenth-grade girls, broken bones occurred three times more often if they drank any kind of soda on a regular basis, and cola drinkers broke bones *five times* as often.

Finally, you would be wise not to drink decaf coffee, as the process of removing the caffeine involves chemicals that may be more harmful than the caffeine that is removed.

VARIETIES OF WATER

Distilled and Reverse-Osmosis Water

Although distilled water is completely pure, the distillation process removes essential and trace minerals that are critical to maintaining proper cell nutrition, and act as important electrical and energy conductors in the body. Because the body is 70 percent water, it's essentially an electrical field that depends on water-based fluids to convey information to the nervous system and organ cells. Since distilled water does not contain the minerals necessary to conduct electricity, the body will seek out these important minerals and may leach them from muscles and bones, leading to a variety of aches and pains, and possibly contributing to osteoporosis. These reservations about distilled water also hold true for reverse-osmosis water, which is available at most of the popular grocery-store chains. Reverse-osmosis is a mechanical means used to purify water, which also depletes it of important minerals.

Rural Well Water

In most cases, it's best to avoid drinking and cooking with rural well water. If you live on a farm or in a rural area with a private well, particularly in an agricultural area of the country, it's very important to take note of this recommendation because there could be significant contaminants in the water. Substances such as toxic barnyard waste runoff, residues of agricultural fertilizers, herbicides, pesticides, and a host of pathologic organisms are commonly found in rural well water. These substances, by themselves or in combination, can cause a variety of disorders and ill health conditions.

Municipal Tap Water

There are also health concerns regarding the municipal tap water in cities and towns. In addition to retaining industrial wastes, poisonous heavy metals, and toxic contaminants, tap water also contains chlorine and fluoride. Chlorine is purposely added to municipal water supplies to kill harmful germs—and it does—but it also kills the body's beneficial germs, the normal intestinal bacteria that we all need to live. Fluoride is added to drinking water in many cities and municipalities to prevent cavities in developing teeth. This practice is controversial, however, for reasons that we will discuss in Chapter 10.

Commercial Bottled Water

You might expect that all commercially bottled water is totally safe to drink, but this is not the case. The consumption of bottled water has increased to the extent that some cities, for purely economic reasons, now bottle and sell their *regular* tap water. Many other companies claim their products are from natural springs and artesian wells, but while this may be technically accurate, there is no guarantee that the source of this water is free from harmful contaminants. The commercial water industry is not fully regulated, and some bottled waters may contain known contaminants or potentially harmful chemicals. Therefore, it's a good idea to know the source of the bottled water you are drinking.

Filtered Water

The most practical, least expensive way to ensure that you are getting pure, high-quality water is to use an effective filtration system for drinking and cooking water. The best filters feature dual filtration, with ceramic and carbon-block technology. It's also a good idea to purchase a high-quality shower filter, as chlorine and other toxins can be absorbed into the body through the skin and through inhalation in an enclosed shower. Because chlorine has other harmful effects on the body, it's wise to minimize your time in chlorinated swimming pools or home hot tubs.

It's been estimated that Americans are spending over $20 billion annually on bottled drinking water and water filtration and purification systems for the home, so you are not alone if you participate in this highly recommended health practice.

3. Structure and Function: Exercising and Maintaining Your Body

ike all the body's other systems, your spine and framework need proper nutrition, exercise, avoidance of toxic exposure, and attention to all the other golden rules of good health outlined in this book. Disturbances of the body's framework can disrupt the function of the nervous system, upset the body's harmony, and set the stage for disease and dysfunction. The Golden Rule presented here deals with the maintenance of your body framework and exercise.

SPINAL AND STRUCTURAL HEALTH

If you want good health, you must take care of your spine. If you want a healthy spine, you must take care of your overall health. Structure and function are intimately related. Your skull and spinal column house and protect the most evolved phenomenon in the known universe, the human brain and nervous system, which regulate all other body systems.

Caring, skillful manual therapy for structural disorders can be very valuable in maintaining the integrity of your framework, thereby improving your health. Competent, professional structural care can positively affect conditions such as back pain and related spinal and extremity disorders, aid in stress management, enhance immune-system function, and improve function of all the other body systems. To begin enjoying these benefits, you may wish to select a doctor of chiropractic (D.C.) or a traditional doctor of osteopathy (D.O.). Since approximately 94 percent of all structural care is currently provided by chiropractors, they are the first choice for most people. Chiropractors believe that approximately 70 to 80 percent of all health disorders involve the neuromusculoskeletal system, including conditions that involve the circulatory, digestive, immune, locomotor, nervous, reproductive, and respiratory systems. Chiropractic and other forms of carefully applied manual therapy can be used to prevent ill health, as well.

Having practiced chiropractic for over forty years, I can attest to witnessing and participating in hundreds of healing experiences that seemed like miracles to the grateful patients. Considerable research has documented the benefits of modern, structurally based health care. Forms of manual care that attend to structure and function and the importance of the nervous system in regulating all other body systems is rapidly becoming an important component of mainstream medicine.

Massage

Therapeutic massage also offers tremendous health benefits. It's good for the body, the mind, and the spirit. Massage therapy has been shown to help effectively maintain health, relieve pain, and reduce stress, and an increasing number of benefits are documented each year. Several intriguing studies examining the effects of massage therapy on newborn babies have indicated a higher likelihood of survival among premature infants, and significant improvements in their immune systems.

Massage therapy is complementary with touch-healing systems such as chiropractic, osteopathic manipulation, and physical therapy, and can also be used with acupuncture and other energy-healing techniques. Massage improves circulation, increases lymph flow, mobilizes waste products from the body, reduces nerve tension, relaxes muscles, and relieves pain. Sometimes I wonder whether it might help put an end to divorce if every married person were to give and receive a half-hour massage from his or her spouse every day. Perhaps this is an exaggeration, but if devoted partners could set aside an hour every day in a quiet, secure atmosphere, and practice this form of intimate touching, it would no doubt contribute a great deal to a long-term, loving relationship. To extend the idea, what if every person in the world gave and received a half-hour massage every day? Could this simple act help put an end to violence and even warfare? Interesting idea—and what have we got to lose?

Muscle Stripping

Healthy, relaxed muscles should be soft, firm, and pliable, with a tone similar to the texture of a recently set gelatin dessert. For aches, pains, and stiffness, especially of the hips, knees, and feet, you may practice a simple muscle-stripping technique with a common kitchen rolling pin. Muscle stripping is not the same as massage and is not necessarily meant to feel good while it is taking place. Simply hold the rolling pin by its handles and gently but firmly roll it over the long muscles of your thighs, shins, and calves. You will typically find dense, hard, painful nodules in these heavily used muscle groups, and when you do, it is important to press firmly enough to elicit mild to moderate discomfort. Although the technique can be somewhat uncomfortable, there is no simpler or more effective technique for successfully working out the knots in the long muscles of the body. Immediate relief, renewed strength, and elasticity of the tissues are the usual results, along with improved mobility and stability of the bones and joints these muscles are designed to move.

You may wish to ask your spouse or a good friend to use the rolling pin for muscle stripping on your more difficult-to-reach hamstring, buttock, spine, or shoulder muscles while you are lying in a comfortable position on your abdomen. When stripping the sides and front of your thigh muscles, you may roll up and down. However, on the back of your calf muscles and on your inner thighs, from the knee to the groin, it's best to roll *upward only* in the direction of your heart. This is crucial because there are important large veins in your calf muscles and on the inner thigh, and firmly massaging or stripping downward could potentially damage one-way valves in the veins and impede the flow of blood back to the heart. As long as you take this simple precaution, this form of tissue massage and muscle-stripping can work wonders for the muscles and joints of the lower extremities. A word of caution regarding muscle stripping: If you have a history of blood clots or severe varicose veins, it is important to consult your doctor prior to performing deep-tissue massage or muscle-stripping techniques, whether by hand or with a rolling pin.

EXERCISE AND STRETCHING PROGRAMS

What about exercise programs? The time-honored expression "use it or lose it" is right on the mark. There's no question that the body requires substantial movement and physical activity to remain healthy and functional, but the types of movement, and the actual amount of physical exertion required is still subject to some debate. As an example, in addition to regular work and recreational activity, the safest and most effective exercises for many people may not be regular exercises at all. Exercise usually implies that you are using, or loading, your muscles. When you are engaged in athletics, performing manual labor, working out, or using your muscles during recreational activities, you are loading them, which causes them to shorten. In most cases, the most frequently used muscles in your body are already too tight and too short so, in this instance, the best exercise routine would be a program of stretching. Gradual, progressive elongation and s-t-r-e-t-c-h-i-n-g of the muscle fibers can work wonders in restoring oxygen and dissipating toxic waste products. I recommend Robert and Jean Anderson's well-illustrated book *Stretching* to learn more about this.

Walking

Go for walks. Taking walks by yourself gives you an opportunity to commune with nature and use the time for personal reflection. Walking regularly with a friend or loved one is excellent, too—for one thing, knowing you have someone to accompany you can improve your exercise discipline, regardless of the weather or other distractions. Although walking in urban or suburban areas is acceptable if you have no alternative, walking in the woods, around a lake, or on the seashore is better, if you can manage it. There really is no set length of time for which you should walk, but keep in mind that any amount of time spent walking is a good investment in your cardiovascular health and a valuable addition to any daily exercise routine.

Running

Running and jogging may be appropriate for some people, but you should pursue these more intense forms of exercise only if your body is well-balanced and structurally and mechanically sound. Even when your bones and joints are in good condition, you should run or jog only on level, shock-absorbent surfaces, such as groomed, grassy parks; playgrounds; and woodland paths. I can't emphasize enough the importance of choosing groomed surfaces, as it's very easy to accidentally step in a hole on a non-groomed surface and risk severe ankle or knee sprain, or disabling fractures. Avoid prolonged running on cement sidewalks, hardwood floors, or blacktop highways, because these surfaces create more shock for the body's joints. The local high school cinder track may be the best surface for running because it's specially designed to absorb shock and, when properly maintained, it's free of holes and uneven surfaces that can cause slips, trips, and falls.

Shoes

Whether you'll be walking, jogging, or running for exercise, be sure to wear the correct shoes. The most common error in purchasing shoes is buying shoes that are too wide or too short. If your shoes seem to wear out prematurely, or if you experience arch or leg cramps; blisters, calluses, or corns; leg, hip, and low-back pain; foot pain; redness from friction; or shin splints, it's possible that your athletic shoes do not fit your feet properly. It may surprise you to learn that most athletic tennis shoes are available only in medium width (size D for men, and B for women), so while about 80 percent of the population can fit into these medium-width shoes, people with narrow feet or wide feet need to be especially concerned about getting shoes that fit properly. Consult a knowledgeable sales-person, and invest in a few pair of extraordinarily good shoes because, when it comes to your feet, you deserve only the best. Excellent shoes are a practical health investment. By purchasing only premium quality, properly fitting shoes, you will own fewer pairs, but you will save money in the long run as the top-notch shoes will last longer and be much better for your health. New Balance is one American shoe company that manufactures and markets athletic shoes in all widths. For further information, consult their website at www.newbalance.com. In addition, it's a good idea to remember that high-impact running causes even the best shoes to break down, so you should replace them regularly, even if they don't show signs of wear.

Women should limit high heels to special occasions. There are many fash-ionable alternatives for everyday wear, so when you go shoe shopping, leave vanity at the door. Your feet *and* the rest of your body—including the expres-sion on your face—will be glad you did.

Aerobic Exercise

What is the role of aerobic exercise in maintaining body structure? The two most important muscles in your body are your heart and diaphragm, and they cannot benefit from an exercise program unless they are challenged by an activity that increases the heart's contraction (pulse) and the breathing (respiration) rates. Aerobic exercise is physically demanding enough to increase your heart and breathing rates by at least 20 percent. The average resting adult heart and breath-ing rate is about seventy-two pulse beats (contractions) and sixteen breaths per minute. Therefore, for an exercise to be considered aerobic, you need to increase your heart rate to about eighty-six contractions per minute and your breathing rate to about twenty breaths per minute. For best results, try to fit twenty min-utes of aerobic exercise into your physical-conditioning routine at least three times a week.

The next best general exercise after walking is probably swimming. Even if you are not a good swimmer, you can stay in the shallow end and have a fun workout. This is especially true if you have access to a chlorine-free area for swimming, as the chlorine in swimming pools poses its own health hazard. Walking and swimming are both aerobic and quadrilateral forms of exercise, meaning that you use both your arms and legs symmetrically and rhythmically. Other recommended aerobic and quadrilateral exercises include most team sports, rollerblading, cross-country skiing, snowshoeing, and most forms of dance. Can you picture yourself dancing with your sweetie across a meadow in the moonlight? Now there's a great way to get your heart rate going!

Weight Training

If you decide to incorporate weight training into your exercise routine, begin with the assistance of a well-trained professional who can show you the proper way to use the equipment. Then you can gradually increase the intensity of your workouts. It's important to remember, however, that a *balanced approach* to exercise is critical, because weight training too often focuses more on physical appearance than on balanced structural integrity.

PREVENTING SPINAL INJURIES

Your spine is the most significant of your body's mechanical structures and is especially deserving of your appreciation and attention. According to the Occupational Safety & Health Administration (OSHA), approximately 85 percent of Americans will have a temporarily disabling injury or disorder of the spine during their working lifetime. Many of these injuries will leave permanent residual pain, and some will result in total, permanent disability. If you have been challenged by recurrent back problems, ask a doctor who specializes in spine disorders for information to help you prevent further injury or to help you cope with chronic symptoms. Fortunately, most back conditions are due to structural malfunctions rather than life-threatening bone, joint, muscle, or organ disease. Once serious disease has been ruled out, structurally related back problems are best treated by manual techniques and attention to nutrition, weight management, hydration, and lifestyle. I highly recommend watching the colorful and entertaining videotape produced by Comprehensive Loss Management, Inc., entitled *Back in Step: The Road to Recovery from Back Pain* by occupational therapist Michael Melnik, M.S., OTR. *Back in Step* will help you gain practical insights regarding safer and more comfortable ways of going about your day, including sitting, standing, lifting, sleeping, kitchen and bathroom activities, child care, yard work, driving, and recreational activities. Even if you have never experienced serious back pain, you will find this program valuable to keep your body healthy and strong.

For employers interested in helping their employees prevent work-related injuries, I recommend an excellent series of education materials also produced by Comprehensive Loss Management, Inc. *Blueprints for Safety,* their training manual, is also available online at www.clmi-training.com.

SUMMARY

It is generally agreed that people should engage in at least *one hour* of physical activity every day. Physical activity includes virtually everything that involves movement and physical exertion. If you are typically more active, the physical work you do combined with recreational activities you enjoy could be just the workout you need to stay in shape. If you are not very active in your everyday life, getting more exercise could be a matter of consistently choosing to take the stairs instead of the elevator where you work.

Don't assume that you have to become an athlete or an aerobics instructor to remain physically fit. Start by following the guidelines in this chapter. Your *attitude* toward maintaining the gift of your physical ability is key to structural and functional health. The single most significant reason why older people enter assisted living facilities and nursing homes is because of disorders of the neuro-musculoskeletal system that prevent them from being able to perform the activities of daily living, such as bathing, dressing, eating, and going to the bathroom; it is not because of cancer, diabetes, heart disease, or some other major organ failure. So, providing thoughtful care for your body's structure will reward you with a lifetime of comfortable, efficient functioning and allow your candle to burn brightly until it's time to go on to greater adventures.

4. Alkalinity and Acidity: The Right Ratio for Your Body

his Golden Rule of good health has to do with the acid/alkaline ratio of your body chemistry. Alkalinity and acidity refer to the pH of the fluids in and around all the cells in your body. A solution with a pH of 7.00 is neutral, one with a pH of more than 7.0 is alkaline, and one with a pH lower than 7.0 is acidic. Under the best conditions, your salivary pH, which mirrors the pH of the fluid bathing all your tissue cells, should be in the alkaline range of 7.0–7.5, with an ideal of 7.4. Every moment you are alive, your body must maintain a 7.3–7.5 pH in the blood. For people who consume a predominantly acid-forming diet or live a stressful lifestyle, the body must continually buffer the blood by using stored alkaline-forming substances—including calcium and other minerals in muscle and bone—in order to maintain this pH. Doing this disturbs the electrochemical balances in the body, overtaxes the system, and results in tissue breakdown, aging of cells, and eventual disease.

ALKALINITY

Keep your body's chemistry *alkaline*. Alkaline-producing foods, which include most fruits and vegetables, leave a digested ash where most of the elements that are beneficial—calcium, magnesium, potassium, and sodium—are positively charged ions. The residual ash of acid-producing foods, such as dairy products, grains (including wheat), meats, and sweets, contains a greater number of negatively charged ions, including chlorine, iodine, phosphorus, and sulfur. This is important to note because infectious viruses can live in an acid environment, but not in an alkaline one. People who keep their bodies in a predominantly alkaline state also have a reduced risk of developing degenerative and inflammatory conditions such as arthritis, cancer, and heart disease.

A simple but highly effective way to help keep your body chemistry alkaline is to squeeze the juice of one-half of a ripe lemon in a glass of water upon rising in the morning. Sip the drink slowly while going through your morning routine. Throughout the day, for lunch, midday snacks, and dinner, keep your body chemistry balanced by predominantly eating and drinking alkaline-forming foods and juices. Doing so will help prevent colds, flu, and other infectious diseases, as well as degenerative and inflammatory conditions.

The following alkaline-forming foods should comprise 80 percent of your diet. Acid-forming foods should provide the remaining 20 percent.

Alkaline-Forming Fruits and Fruit Juices

Apples, apricots, bananas (ripe), cantaloupe, cherries, currants, dates, figs, grapes, grapefruit, guava, honeydew, kiwi, kumquats, lemons, limes, mangos, muskmelon, nectarines, oranges, papaya, passionfruit, peaches, pears, pineapple, raisins, raspberries, strawberries, tangerines, and watermelon

Alkaline-Forming Vegetables and Vegetable Juices

Artichokes, asparagus, bamboo shoots, beets, broccoli, Brussels sprouts, cabbage, carrots, cauliflower, celery, collards, corn (sweet), cucumbers, eggplant, endive, escarole (a form of lettuce), flaxseed, green beans, horseradish, kale, kelp, kohlrabi, leeks, lettuce, lima beans, mushrooms, mustard greens, okra, onions, parsley, parsnips, peas, peppers, potatoes, pumpkin, radishes, rhubarb, rutabaga, sauerkraut, seaweed, soybeans and soybean products, spinach, squash, Swiss chard, tomatoes (ripe), turnips, water chestnuts, watercress, and yams

Alkaline-Forming Nuts

Almonds, chestnuts, and coconut (fresh)

Alkaline-Forming Oils

Almond, avocado, canola, castor, coconut, corn, flax, olive, safflower, sesame, soy, and sunflower

Alkaline-Forming Sugars and Sweeteners

Dried sugar-cane juice, honey (raw, unpasteurized), and molasses

Alkaline-Forming Herbal Teas

Alfalfa, clover, comfrey, ginseng, mint, raspberry, sage, spearmint, and strawberry

Alkaline-Forming Seasonings

Anise, bay leaves, basil, caraway seed, cayenne pepper, celery seed, chives, cider vinegar (raw, unpasteurized), cinnamon, cloves, curry powder, dill, fennel seed, garlic, ginger, marjoram, nutmeg, oregano, paprika, rosemary, sage, sea salt, and vanilla extract

ACIDITY

Acid-forming foods should be eaten in moderation, keeping alkaline-forming foods dominant in the diet As described above, a diet of 80 percent alkaline-forming foods and 20 percent acid-forming foods is ideal to maintain good health and prevent disease.

Common Acid-Forming Foods

Many bean family foods, including, garbanzo, kidney, lentil, mung, navy, pinto, red, and white beans

Most breads, cereals, and pastas

Cranberries and cranberry juice

Most dairy products, including butter, cheese, cream, ice cream, milk (cow and goat), whey, and yogurt

Eggs and custards

Meats of all species, including fish and seafoods

Most grains, including barley, buckwheat, corn meal, oats, rice, rye, and wheat

Many nuts, including, Brazil nuts, cashews, filberts, macadamia nuts, peanuts, pecans, pistachios, and walnuts

Most sugars and sweeteners, including artificial sweeteners, beet sugar, cane sugar (white processed), fructose, honey (processed or pasteurized), maple syrup, and milk sugar

Acid-Forming Substances to Avoid

Alcohol products

Black tea

Caffeine, including coffee

Candy

Carbonated beverages and any soft drinks

Corn syrup

Drugs, prescription and over the counter

Many cosmetics

Ketchup

Mayonnaise

Margarine

Any hydrogenated or partially hydrogenated oil that contains trans-fatty acids, such as shortenings, cooking or deep-frying oil, and salad oils

Refined white flour in bread, cookies, doughnuts, pastries, pies, sweet rolls, and so forth

Refined white sugar in pre-sweetened cereals

Tobacco products

White processed (distilled) vinegar

Some of the most harmful acid-forming substances are drugs—in fact, 98 percent of all prescription and over-the-counter drugs promote acid-forming reactions in the body. Of course, certain drugs can have critical, lifesaving value, but many also have potentially life-threatening side effects. Physicians are wise to prescribe drugs selectively.

Excessive consumption of acid-forming foods, beverages, and other products can result in a variety of infectious and degenerative diseases. For more on the importance of balancing your intake of alkaline and acidic foods and other products, read Dr. Theodore Baroody's book *Alkalize or Die,* which discusses foods, food groups, food preparation, and recipes for maintaining the proper alkaline/acid ratio.

NECTERRA PLUS

Necterra Plus is a concentrated blend of nature's most perfect whole foods that has powerful alkalizing, anti-aging, and antioxidant effects. Taken daily, it is an excellent way to help keep your body chemistry alkaline. The ingredients in Necterra Plus include, in descending order: organically grown apple cider vinegar; raw, unpasteurized honey; bee pollen; royal jelly; wheat, barley, and rye grasses; alfalfa; soy lecithin; spirulina; pectin apple fiber; sprouted barley malt; brown rice bran; pineapple powder pectin; Nova Scotia dulse; fructooligosaccharides; chlorella; beet juice powder; oat and rye grass powders; Siberian ginseng powder; grapeseed and peppermint leaf extracts; acerola juice powder; licorice root; rhubarb juice powder; aloe vera; ginkgo biloba; and ginger root and bilberry leaf powders.

Necterra Plus is also fortified with an exclusive blend of more than seventy essential and trace minerals derived from a healing clay deposit that was once an ancient seabed. Because this rare, mineral-rich clay deposit has been exposed to thousands of years of geothermal activity, it has extraordinary healing properties. Indeed, the clay has been used by people of native cultures for centuries, both externally and internally. In addition, Necterra Plus has electromagnetic frequencies in its liquid mineral clay suspension that react well with the body's own electrical nature.

Adding Necterra Plus to fruit smoothies or stirring two tablespoons into a glass of water or juice to drink with meals instead of coffee, tea, or soft drinks is an easy way to benefit from this nutrient-rich substance. It can also be used as a base for a delicious, healthy salad dressing. I highly recommend Necterra Plus for virtually anyone who wants to increase natural energy and achieve optimal health. This is a product that could, as the old saying goes, add years to your life

A High-Energy Alkalizing Fruit-and-Nut Smoothie Recipe

An excellent and tasty way to achieve alkaline body chemistry and to take in the carbohydrates, proteins, amino acids, essential oils, fiber, minerals, raw food enzymes, and vitamins you need for optimal health is to start your day with a fresh-fruit-and-nut smoothie. I recommend this over the traditional American acid-forming, artery-clogging breakfast of bacon, ham, sausage, fried eggs, fried potatoes, several cups of strong coffee, white toast or sweet roll, all polished off with a cigarette or two for the road. Sound familiar?

Here is the recipe for my personal favorite smoothie. Simply blend the following ingredients together for a delicious treat. Remember to always use organically grown products when possible.

Two or three ripe bananas

A handful of fully ripened strawberries, raspberries, or blueberries (fresh frozen in winter months)

One or two kiwis

A small handful of raw, unsalted almonds

Two heaping tablespoons of ground flaxseed powder

A slice of watermelon, honeydew, or muskmelon, or a bit of each—whatever you have on hand

One or two slices of fresh apricot, nectarine, peach, or pineapple

For variety, occasionally a few dates, figs, or prunes

One or two teaspoons of Udo's Perfected Oil Blend

Two or three tablespoons of Necterra Plus

One or two packets of Knox Gelatine, which protects your cartilage, collagen, and joints, and is also good for your hair, nails, and skin

You may vary any of the above to suit your taste. The quantities above will make a full blender (30 ounces) of nutrient-rich, anti-aging, antioxidant, whole raw food that will generously serve two or three people. It only takes about ten minutes to prepare, and the ingredients total about $5.00.

Smoothies are fun, delicious, nutritious, and easy to make—overall a great way to help keep your body chemistry alkaline and your systems operating at peak performance. Making a fruit-and-nut smoothie a daily habit can become a very important step in preventing disease and preserving your health.

A word of caution: If you have diabetes or moderate to severe hypoglycemia, you should take your individual sugar limit into consideration because this recipe could contain an excess of carbohydrates.

and life to your years. Necterra Plus is available through NuHealth Wellness. You can visit the company's website at nuhealthwellness.com.

MONITOR YOUR ALKALINITY/ACIDITY THROUGH SALIVA

An easy, accurate, and inexpensive way to monitor your body's pH is to use standard pH paper to test your saliva. If it's not available at your pharmacy or health food store, you can ask them to order it for you or order it yourself. My preferred brand is by Vaxa—Natural Solutions for Life's Challenges. Call 1-800-248-8292 and ask for the Medical pH-Test Strips, or contact them at their website: www.Vaxa.com. The strips come in 30 count and 100 count and cost approximately $12 and $18 respectively. The paper indicates pH ranges between 1 (very acidic) and 14 (very alkaline).

Follow the directions on the label. Most pH testing paper has a limited shelf life, so purchase it in small quantities. You can extend its life by keeping the strips tightly sealed in the original container, and storing it in a dry, cool place away from heat or direct sunlight. The test is most accurate first thing in the morning, prior to bathing and before any significant physical activity. For the test to be accurate, wait about two hours after eating, chewing gum, sucking on breath mints, or ingesting anything. Swallow any saliva in your mouth, then place one end of the paper strip beneath your tongue, where there is a rich supply of new saliva, and hold it for just a few seconds. Remove the strip and note the color you observe will correspond to the pH numbers. If the test paper reveals a pH of six or less, which is more acidic, this underscores your need for the dietary, lifestyle, and attitudinal information outlined throughout this book. You may also want to test your pH between meals and before bedtime. Don't forget to record your test results each time you measure your pH. Until you have established a pattern that sustains the desired alkaline state, you should probably test two, three, even four times a day. Performing this simple pH testing will give you a reasonably accurate assessment of your body's acid/alkaline chemistry, which can help guide your ongoing food choices and lifestyle decisions.

5. Medicinal Wonder Foods

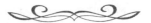

his Golden Rule concerns your appreciation for foods that have medicinal properties. Most of the foods described in this chapter are available in the produce and natural foods section of most traditional grocery stores and farmers' markets. Finding some of the less common items may require a trip to an organic food co-op or a health food store. Almost all traditional foods are considered safe for general consumption. However, if you have questions or concerns regarding whether a particular food, herb, oil, or botanical product is right for you, it is wise to consult a knowledgeable healthcare professional. He or she can, for example, answer your questions regarding recommended dosages and address your concerns about possible interactions with any medications you may be taking or any food sensitivities or allergies you may have.

WONDER FOODS

No doubt, you have heard of wonder drugs that have been credited with significant breakthroughs in advancing health and saving lives. Certainly, some of these agents deserve our respect and recognition, particularly in emergency and crisis situations, and for thoughtful use in managing advanced, irreversible disease states. However, the wondrous healing properties of dozens and dozens of whole foods and whole-food derivatives, herbs, botanical plants, aromatic and essential oils are now being rediscovered.

Garlic

Probably no household food has more documentation regarding its remarkable healing properties than garlic. Often described as a healing elixir and restorer of youth, garlic is well-known throughout the world for its germ-fighting, anti-aging, antioxidant, and body-cleansing effects. For infections of any kind, garlic is sometimes referred to as nature's penicillin. Available literature provides us with information on everything to do with garlic, from curing the common cold and stopping the morning sickness of pregnancy to preventing many forms of cancer.

Perhaps garlic's greatest benefit is its ability to prevent vascular disorders such as blood clots that can cause heart attack and strokes, and hardening of the arteries. It has also been proven effective in lowering blood pressure and blood cholesterol levels. Garlic can also improve the body's ability to absorb B vitamins. In particular, it can increase the absorption of vitamin C up to ten times. If you don't already know about the wonders of garlic, I recommend you learn about its many health-enhancing and illness-preventing aspects and begin to use it daily.

Garlic's characteristic odor can be a problem if you are in the close company of others on a daily basis. However, garlic perles available in health food and grocery stores contain all the active healing properties of fresh garlic cloves, without the pungent odor. I recommend KWAI and Kyolic, both of which are available in any health food store, supermarket, or pharmacy. For maximum value, I recommended using garlic throughout the day, two perles with each meal, rather than in large quantities all at once.

Onion

Another wonder food, closely related to garlic, is the onion. As first cousins in the food family, onions have preventive and healing effects similar to garlic and can be added to your diet for variety and taste. Raw onion is best, but including cooked onion in your diet is also beneficial.

Udo's Choice Perfected Oil Blend

This ingenious blend of essential oils combines certified organic flax, sesame, sunflower, and evening primrose oils; rice bran; oat bran; and rosemary to provide the ideal balance of omega-3, omega-6, and omega-9 essential fatty acids. For this reason, it is a highly effective brain food that helps relieve depression, prevents blood clots and plaque buildup in blood vessels, and facilitates proper electrical and nerve activity. For more information on the important health benefits of essential oils, I recommend Dr. Udo Erasmus' excellent book *Fats That Heal, Fats That Kill.*

Udo's Choice Perfected Oil Blend is available in the refrigerated section of most health foods stores.

Cider Vinegar

In recent years, over 10,000,000 people have purchased Paul and Patricia Bragg's book *Apple Cider Vinegar—Miracle Health System,* which describes the dozens of healing benefits of apple cider vinegar. Rich in enzymes and minerals, this known antibiotic and germ fighter improves digestion and the assimilation of nutrients, and helps the body eliminate toxins. Apple cider vinegar is also great for the skin—a known antioxidant that helps maintain the integrity of tissue cells, thereby slowing the aging process.

Raw Non-Pasteurized Honey

Honey is an instant energy food. It has all the essential minerals necessary for life, seven of the B-complex vitamins, amino acids, enzymes, and other vital factors, and it helps the body maintain its proper alkaline/acid balance. Once honey is processed and pasteurized, a procedure requiring excessive heating, much of its nutritional value is lost, so for maximum health benefits, it's best to use raw, natural, unprocessed honey. It's important to note that children under age two should not be given non-pasteurized honey because their immune systems may not be able to withstand any harmful microorganisms. Buy it raw, before it gets to the processors. Find a respected local beekeeper and become a favorite customer.

Barley Grass, Oat Grass, Rye Grass, and Wheat Grass

Energy- and nutrient-rich antioxidant grasses have been used for medicinal purposes for thousands of years. Harvested in the very early stages of their development, they contain large amounts of chlorophyll, and are natural cleansers and detoxifiers. The juice of barley grass alone contains eleven times the calcium of cow's milk, nearly six times the iron of spinach, seven times the vitamin C of oranges, and is also rich in vitamin B_{12}.

Alfalfa

Alfalfa is extraordinarily rich in vitamins and minerals. Its roots go deep—up to eighteen feet down in the earth—so that it can extract many essential and trace minerals other plants cannot. As a bowel cleanser and natural diuretic, alfalfa aids in the prevention and treatment of urinary tract infections, arthritis, bladder, kidney, and prostate disorders. And it's another exceptional food to help keep the body chemistry alkaline, as well as toxin-free.

SUPPLEMENTAL NUTRIENTS
Bee Pollen

Many consider bee pollen to be nature's most perfect food. There are twenty-two important nutrients in bee pollen, and it has five to seven times more protein than beef. It is truly a wonder food and one of the most effective immune-system builders known. Caution is in order, however, if you are allergic to bee stings, because pollen could trigger a serious allergic reaction.

Royal Jelly

Royal jelly is made by worker bees for the queen bee, and it's another of nature's perfect foods. While the queen bee produces twice her weight in eggs every day and lives for approximately five years, the worker bees who provide the royal jelly for her live only about three months. Royal jelly is a rich source of all the B vitamins, minerals, and amino acids, and has antimicrobial properties. It is known to be beneficial in the prevention and treatment of a wide variety of ailments, including lung, liver, pancreas, stomach, skin, and kidney disorders. It also assists in healing bone fractures and supports the immune system. Although much research has focused on the significant health benefits of royal jelly, about 20 percent of this incredible compound still remains a total mystery.

Soy Lecithin

Lecithin performs an astonishing range of vital functions affecting human health and well-being. It is often considered a brain food due to its balancing and nourishing effects on the entire nervous system. But the benefits don't end there. Lecithin helps reduce cholesterol, prevents fats from accumulating on the walls of arteries, and plays a part in dissolving fatty plaque that may already be clogging the arteries. For a variety of health reasons, I recommend that every person in the world consume soy lecithin daily.

Spirulina

Spirulina is 60 percent protein—making it the world's most concentrated source of protein—and contains all eight essential amino acids, which makes it a complete protein. It is the world's best known vegetable source of vitamin B_{12} and, additionally, has concentrations of A, B_1, B_2, B_6, D, E, and K. Spirulina is also high in essential fatty acids.

Chlorella

Chlorella is a microscopic, green freshwater plant that contains more than twenty different vitamins, and minerals, plus beta-carotene. It's also rich in natural chlorophyll, iodine, iron, lysine, and zinc, and contains more vitamin B_{12}—a nutrient often lacking in many vegetarian diets—than liver.

Ginseng

You've probably heard of ginseng, a popular herb found in America, China, and Russia. In China, it has been used for over 7,000 years and is best known for its medicinal elements and its rejuvenation properties. The list of health benefits this herb provides is nothing short of remarkable. These benefits include the prevention and management of the following: stomach and lung disorders; arthritis and other inflammatory conditions; glandular malfunctions; physical and mental exhaustion; and sexual dysfunctions. I recommend finding out more about this natural wonder food and adding it to your supplementation program.

Aloe Vera

Aloe is variously described as the medicine plant and the plant of immortality. It is an extraordinary food plant that can be used externally for the treatment of burns, infections, parasites, and wounds, and is used internally for the prevention and treatment of colitis, digestive disorders, and ulcers. And if that weren't enough, aloe is great for improving circulation; aids gallbladder, kidney, and liver functions; and helps maintain the immune system and detoxify the body.

Ginkgo Biloba

Ginkgo biloba is one of the best-researched herbs in the world. In the last thirty years, more than 300 studies have shown that this anti-aging, antioxidant, natural whole food is beneficial for a wide range of health concerns throughout the body. It has great value to the vascular system, particularly in the brain, and therefore is useful in the prevention and treatment of conditions in which circulation to the brain is less than optimal, such as Alzheimer's disease. Additionally, ginkgo can improve mood, enhance memory, increase alertness, and restore energy. *Precautionary Note:* If you are using any medication that contains the blood thinner coumadin, it would be a good idea to talk to a holistically oriented practitioner about the use of ginkgo biloba, and at the same time discuss any other drugs you may be taking for possible contraindications.

ADDITIONAL WONDER FOODS

Asparagus, avocado, bone meal, brewer's yeast, broccoli, cabbage and cabbage juice, cayenne pepper, celery, cherries and pure cherry juice, fish oils, flaxseed, okra, grapes and pure grape juice, papaya, parsley, pumpkin seeds, rutin (buckwheat is a good source), sesame seeds, spinach, strawberries, sunflower seeds, and wheat germ oil. All of these whole, natural, widely available foods are known to contain significant healing properties. Each has its own unique bio-chemical makeup and may or may not be valuable as a curative agent for your particular health condition. However, since they have curative value for some conditions, it's only logical that including them in your diet may well have significant preventive effects.

If you are using foods for their specific medicinal agents, choose certified organic food sources. And remember that the best medicines are those you take to help you stay well—to paraphrase the Father of Medicine, Hippocrates, who said, "Food is your best medicine and the best foods are the best medicine."

Still not convinced about the relationship of foods to health? Consider the following: In a recent study that compared the diets and health of 1,271 people, researchers at the Harvard School of Public Health found that strawberry lovers were 70 percent less likely to develop cancer than those who seldom ate this extraordinary medicinal food.

6. Nutritional Supplements

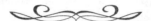

Can the average person maintain vibrant health, energy, and vitality without taking vitamin and mineral supplements? In an ideal world, the answer would be yes, because it would be possible to obtain all the nutrients the body needs from fresh, whole foods. However, between the depletion of nutrient-rich farm soils and our very busy lifestyles that preclude growing our own foods, this is simply not possible or practical, so supplementing with the appropriate nutrients is recommended.

To get the maximum benefits from your supplementation program, I recommend reading up on the subject, and perhaps consulting an alternative or complementary practitioner who has access to the latest research on vitamins, minerals, herbs, enzymes, botanical medicines, homeopathic preparations, and dietary lifestyle. Obviously, you know your own body, mind, and spirit better than anyone on earth. You know your symptoms, habits, addictions, body rhythms, and the other factors that make you unique. By doing your own reading and research, you can greatly aid any professionals you may initially consult when you start your supplementation program.

SPECIFIC VITAMINS AND MINERALS

"All things in moderation" is a logical axiom for healthy living, and can certainly be said for the use of some vitamins and minerals. Unless you are in the highly unusual circumstance of having been diagnosed with a primary nutritional deficiency disease, it is unlikely that large quantities of individual nutritional supplements would benefit you. In fact, it is possible to overdose on certain supplements, particularly the oil-soluble vitamins A, D, E, and K. In most cases, the body is able to discard nutrients it cannot utilize, but intentionally overloading on such substances places extra stress on the liver and kidneys, which could create imbalances.

Vitamin C

Vitamin C is probably purchased more than any other nutritional supplement. This is certainly understandable when you consider its incredible value in protecting against devastating diseases, such as arthritis, cancer, heart disease, immune system disorders, and infections. Smokers and tobacco users, in particular, must pay special attention to consuming foods rich in vitamin C every day because nicotine destroys this nutrient. In fact, the majority of smokers would benefit greatly from a high-quality natural vitamin C supplement because it repairs connective tissue and is also an excellent anti-stress nutrient, as well as a powerful antioxidant. Since vitamin C cannot be stored in the human body, it's important to replenish the nutrient every day.

Make sure the vitamin C supplement you purchase contains bioflavonoids. In nature, vitamin C always has bioflavonoids, sometimes referred to as vitamin P. Many claim that the inexpensive, widely available, ascorbic acid is vitamin C, but others refer to it as synthetic vitamin C because it is lacking in bioflavonoids. Vitamin C with rose hips is an excellent natural form of the nutrient with the bioflavonoid component intact. Although a bit more expensive, and sold mainly in health food stores, the difference between vitamin C with rose hips and other, inferior products can be significant, so it's well worth the investment.

Vitamin E

As a physician, if I had only one vitamin supplement to offer my patients, it would probably be vitamin E because, in addition to the dozens of benefits it provides on its own, the nutrient makes all the other vitamins work more effectively. As a powerful antioxidant, vitamin E is an anti-aging factor and does wonders for the cardiovascular system, including the heart, blood, and lymph vessels throughout the body. When you purchase vitamin E, look for the words d-alpha-tocopherol acetate or acid succinate on the label to be sure you are getting the most potent form of the nutrient. If you look carefully at the label of any inexpensively priced vitamin E capsules, you will see it does not say d-alpha-tocopherol acetate, it says *dl*-alpha-tocopherol acetate, a synthetic substitute for the real thing. Capsules containing d-alpha-tocopherol are more expensive than other types of vitamin E, but well worth the difference in cost. My preferred brand of vitamin E, Key-E Kaps, is manufactured by the Carlson Company (Key-E Kaps).

Calcium

Almost everyone knows the importance of essential and trace minerals for good health, especially elements such as calcium. This critical mineral is required for at least eighteen major functions in the body, including blood buffering, bone and joint formation and repair, brain and nerve function, and muscle work. Calcium deficiency can cause symptoms such as fatigue, muscle cramping, and nervousness, and increase the chance of developing conditions such as osteoporosis, and a tendency to suffer fractures, joint injuries, and muscle strain.

Recent studies indicate that calcium plays a significant role in preventing serious diseases such as arthritis, cancer, and heart disease, by helping to keep the body chemistry alkaline. Adults should consume between 1,500 and 3,000 milligrams (mg) of calcium per day. Large individuals who are athletic or work at physically demanding jobs require more calcium than workers who are less active. Women who are pregnant or breastfeeding should increase their calcium intake, as well as those women who have had one or both ovaries surgically removed.

Excellent calcium sources are dairy products, fresh salmon, leafy green vegetables, canned mackerel and sardines, and nuts and seeds, especially sesame seeds. Calcium is absorbed best if it's taken when the stomach is acid, and is therefore most effective when taken before meals. If a calcium supplement is taken at night, when the body's supply of the nutrient is depleted, it has the added advantage of promoting sleep. Avoid antacids, such as *Tums,* as a dietary source of calcium since these products contain only the oyster-shell form of the mineral, which is not easily assimilated by the body and can cause allergic reactions in some individuals. Calcium citrate is the recommended form of the mineral because it is very effectively utilized by the body.

Can drinking a generous amount of milk every day supply enough calcium to meet an adult's nutritional requirements? Whole milk should probably be cut from the diet because of its fat content, and replaced with skim milk, which provides the same amount of calcium. In general, milk is not the best choice as a source of calcium, especially since the minerals and other nutrients in milk are readily available in other foods, and nature intended it only as a food for infant mammals. As you are probably aware, when a baby suckles or drinks milk and swallows it, the sweet liquid—with the aid of certain naturally occurring enzymes—rapidly forms into curds, or milk solids, for digestion in the stomach and upper digestive tract. As children grow into adulthood, the enzyme required for the formation of milk solids is no longer present in the body, causing many adults to have difficulty digesting milk. But although the need for this form of liquid food ceases, humans seem to be the only mammals who choose not to wean themselves from milk and, instead, continue drinking it into adulthood.

If you are a milk lover, it's also important to recognize that commercial milk is always homogenized. This means that the fat globules contained in milk have been broken up into ultra-microscopic particles that may actually increase the potential for the clogging of blood vessels and hardening of the arteries, thus contributing to arteriosclerosis, heart attack, and stroke. In addition, commercial milk is always pasteurized to kill germs, but this also destroys all of its valuable enzymes, reducing its original food value. While I am not personally opposed to drinking milk, I believe it's important to take all of these facts into consideration. If you love milk and it agrees with your digestion, then go ahead and enjoy it. It's still a great source of calcium, protein, and other vitamins and minerals, after all.

Current farming practices have resulted in our nation's soils becoming depleted of nutrients needed for good health, and this has, in turn, resulted in foods raised in these soils becoming depleted of these necessary nutrients. Thus, if you feel your diet is not providing adequate amounts of calcium, taking calcium supplements may be critical to your health. Keep in mind, however, that calcium supplements should contain vitamin D and magnesium for maximum absorption by the body. I also suggest taking phosphorous-free calcium supplements, especially if you frequently enjoy meat, bread, and soft drinks, all of which are rich in phosphorous. Too much phosphorous can contribute to osteoporosis. Soft drinks contain phosphoric acid. Remember the Harvard study described earlier which found that women athletes who drank soda experienced three to five times more fractures than those who did not drink soda. The body requires two calcium ions for every phosphorous ion, which means that if your diet is already rich in phosphorous, using calcium tablets containing phosphorous perpetuates this imbalance, contributing to the potential for osteoporosis, bone weakening, fractures, muscle cramps, fatigue, and a variety of other calcium- and mineral-deficiency symptoms.

People who have used steroids, such as cortisone or prednisone, are also more prone to demineralization, which can lead to osteoporosis and bone fractures. Caucasians and Asians are more susceptible to osteoporosis than people of African descent. Also, your chance of developing osteoporosis is higher if you have a small bone frame.

Osteoporosis and Menopause

In addition to a lack of physical activity, exercise, sunshine, vitamins D and C, and a deficiency of calcium and magnesium, probably the single most significant cause of bone demineralization in women is an imbalance in the female sex hormones that occurs with the onset of menopause. Doctors often prescribe hormone replacement therapy (HRT) in the form of estrogen and progestin (a synthetic progesterone) to reduce the risk of osteoporosis and alleviate symptoms of menopause such as hot flashes, mood swings, and depression. Unfortunately, this practice has resulted in some serious and disturbing outcomes. Research conducted by the Women's Health Initiative, and reported in a 2002 issue of the *Journal of the American Medical Association,* showed that women who had undergone such therapy actually had increased risks of developing a number of life-threatening illnesses. The study reported, among women who were given HRT, a 26-percent increase in the risk of breast cancer; a 29-percent increase in coronary heart disease (heart attack); a 41-percent increase in strokes, and a 113-percent increase in pulmonary embolism (blood clot in the lung).

A More Natural Approach

Dr. John Lee, a Harvard Medical School graduate with more than thirty years of clinical practice, was perhaps the world's foremost authority on the topic of HRT. Instead of using prescribed estrogen and progestin, Dr. Lee strongly urged women experiencing hormonal imbalance to use natural, plant-derived progesterone that can be applied topically and absorbed through the skin. His research showed significant health benefits from the use of this safe, effective approach to preventing and even reversing osteoporosis. In addition, he showed that estrogen dominance is common in females of all age groups causing a host of symptoms, including acceleration of the aging process; allergies, asthma, hives, and rashes; anxiety; autoimmune disorders such as lupus; breast tenderness; decreased libido; depression; fat deposition around the hips, abdomen, and thighs; fatigue; fibrocystic breast disease; gallbladder disease; hair thinning or loss; headaches; increased risk of blood clots and strokes; infertility; insomnia; irregular menstrual cycles; low blood sugar; memory loss; miscarriage; mood swings; premenstrual syndrome (PMS); skin conditions (such as psoriasis); uterine cancer or fibroids; water retention; and bloating.

For women who may be experiencing symptoms of a hormonal imbalance, I highly recommend Dr. Lee's two books on this timely and important subject: *What Your Doctor May Not Tell You About Menopause: The Breakthrough Book on Natural Progesterone* and *What Your Doctor May Not Tell You About Pre-Menopause: Balance Your Hormones and Your Life From Thirty to Fifty.* Another excellent informational source is *This Is Not Your Mother's Menopause: One Woman's Natural Journey Through Change* by Trisha Posner.

Magnesium

Another very important yet often overlooked mineral is magnesium. It is believed that up to 80 percent of the adult population in the United States is currently deficient in magnesium. While calcium is important for muscle firing and nerve conduction, magnesium is necessary for muscle relaxation. Muscle cramps, spasms, ticks, twitches, shin splints, and even asthma attacks, depression, insomnia, and menstrual cramps can all result from inadequate magnesium intake. The recommended dosage is 5 mg of magnesium per pound of body weight daily. Therefore, if you weigh 150 pounds, you should make sure you're getting a minimum of 450 mg of magnesium every day. Natural sources of magnesium include fresh unsalted almonds, brown rice, leafy green vegetables, legumes (beans and peas), and whole grains.

Sodium Chloride and Potassium

For most people, it is very important to reduce or moderate sodium-chloride (salt) intake and increase potassium intake. Most people consume far more sodium than potassium—up to ten times more, in some cases—but the ideal ratio is twice the amount of potassium to sodium. Common sources of sodium chloride that we often consume in excess are cold cuts, frozen foods, meats, processed foods, salted nuts, sausage, and snack foods such as popcorn, potato chips, and pretzels. To increase your potassium intake to balance your sodium-to-potassium ratio, choose foods such as bananas, dried fruits, fish, molasses, oranges or orange juice, raw vegetables, squash, and sunflower seeds.

If you've been instructed to maintain a low- or no-sodium diet, you'll be happy to know that excellent salt substitutes and seasonings are available. Most of them use potassium chloride as the replacement for sodium chloride and provide the same salt flavor as traditional salt. My personal favorite salt substitute is an herb seasoning sea-salt product known as Herbamare, which is available at most health food stores. In addition to sea-salt minerals, it contains the fresh, organically grown herbs basil, celery leaves, chives, watercress and garden cress, garlic, kelp (a rich source of iodine), leek, lovage, marjoram, onion, parsley, rosemary, and thyme. One precaution should be mentioned for people who no longer consume commercial table salt: because most salt has been iodized (iodine added) for the prevention of iodine deficiency, cutting out table salt entirely may cause a deficiency of this vital nutrient. Iodine deficiency results in thyroid problems and goiter, so people who adopt a low-salt diet must be sure they are getting an adequate iodine intake in order to maintain good health. This is especially true for people living inland from the oceans who are not as likely to consume iodine-rich seafood on a regular basis.

BUYING AND USING MULTIVITAMIN AND -MINERAL SUPPLEMENTS

Be sure your multivitamin and -mineral supplements include naturally occurring, plant-derived, digestive enzymes. Enzymes are absolutely essential for complete breakdown and absorption of nutrients in the digestive tract. Many commercially sold nutritional supplements simply are not fully digestible by the body, making them a waste of money and time. Gelatin-coated capsules, powders, and liquid supplements absorb much more completely and are therefore a significantly better value. This is one of the reasons I recommend Necterra Plus whole foods liquid concentrate by EnTerra. It has a long, established track record of being super-absorbent and therefore of maximum nutritive value.

Time-Release Vitamins and Minerals

It's probably best to avoid most time-release vitamin and mineral supplements. Since there's no guarantee when and where the tablet's active ingredients will be released in the digestive tract, it could expose the body to potential overloads and overwhelm the liver's ability to detoxify the system. This is especially true of niacin. Pregnant women and people with diabetes, gout, stomach ulcers, or liver disease should be aware that large amounts of this nutrient suddenly released into their bloodstreams may overtax their systems, resulting in an inability to properly neutralize it.

ADDITIONAL SUPPLEMENTS FOR GOOD HEALTH

Enzymes

Enzymes are essential to life. They are the catalysts that spark every chemical reaction in the body, and they are necessary for the digestion of food. Incredible numbers of enzymes are needed to keep cells humming vibrantly within their electromagnetic energy fields and, in fact, every cell in the body must manufacture the enzymes needed for its own survival and function. In addition, the body requires enzymes from food sources that it cannot make on its own. Only raw foods, particularly fresh vegetables, fruits, and juices, contain enzymes. When you bake, boil, broil, microwave, roast, steam, stew, can, or pasteurize your food, all the food enzymes are destroyed by the heat. Because so many of us live almost exclusively on cooked, processed, and refined foods, we may require additional enzymes for optimal health. This is particularly true as we grow older because aging reduces the body's ability to manufacture its own enzymes. By adding enzymes to your diet, your food will digest better, you'll have more energy, and you'll experience much less bloating, gas, and indigestion. *Enzyme Nutrition* and *Food Enzymes for Health and Longevity* by Dr. Edward Howell are both excellent books on the subject.

Antioxidants

Antioxidants are foods and food supplements that help to slow or reduce the aging and degeneration process in the body. Alpha-lipoic acid; coenzyme Q_{10}; curcumin; resveratrol from grape skins and seeds; vitamins A, C, and E; and the mineral selenium are particularly well-known antioxidants. As discussed, it's important to eat plenty of fresh fruits, vegetables, seeds, and nuts to attain and preserve optimal health. In addition to being rich in vitamins, minerals, enzymes, and naturally occurring oils, these premium plant foods are the principal sources of antioxidants. Even if your diet is replete with them, it may also help to use supplementary antioxidants.

Flaxseed Benefits Both Men and Women

Recent studies have indicated that ground flaxseed taken daily can provide excellent health benefits for both the male and female reproductive systems. Flaxseeds are a rich source of the nutrients the body needs to manufacture the two most important hormones that enhance the normal function of the uterus, ovaries, and breasts, and protect them from a variety of disorders, including cancer. Many of the hormone-imbalance symptoms described on page 40 can be relieved with this excellent, inexpensive food. These same phytoestrogens, or plant estrogens, help prevent prostate enlargement and prostate cancer in men, especially when taken in combination with herbs such as saw palmetto. Ground flaxseed also helps to lower blood cholesterol, making it important in preventing heart disease and hardening of the arteries; supports liver and gallbladder health, normal bowel function, and bone density; and improves tone and texture of the skin.

You may purchase flaxseed and grind it yourself in a home coffee grinder, or buy it already ground in bulk quantities through your local health food store. When available, choose certified organic flaxseed or ground flaxseed powder. Take two or three heaping tablespoons daily blended in smoothies, stirred into your favorite fruit juices, or sprinkled on breakfast cereals. You can also add flaxseed to your salad dressings or to other seasonings. It will add a pleasant, nutty flavor to all your foods, regardless of how you consume it.

7. Rest and Sleep

I n today's fast-paced, competitive society, many Americans are working or playing longer hours and therefore sleeping less. Indeed it's gotten to the point where sleep deprivation, with its negative consequences for health, has become almost epidemic. The importance of getting adequate sleep cannot be overstated, because it's during this time that the body repairs and heals itself. For most people, getting "enough" sleep means enjoying at least seven to eight hours of restful sleep during each twenty-four-hour period. Quality of sleep is probably more important than quantity because, during the deepest portion of the sleep cycle, the body's tissues and nervous system are repaired and restored. Clearly, it's important to do whatever it takes to increase your chances of sound, deep, uninterrupted sleep, and this means following the Golden Rules outlined in this chapter.

KEYS TO A GOOD NIGHT'S SLEEP

Your Bed and Mattress

There are two things you should freely spend money on—the best pair of shoes and the best set of bedding you can buy—because chances are you will spend the great majority of your future in one or the other. Be extravagant when you choose your bed, mattress, and pillow. You're worth it.

Throughout the years, many of my patients have asked, "Doctor, as a spine specialist, what do you consider the best mattress on the market?" While this question may sound rather simple, its answer can be challenging because different beds and mattresses are required for different shapes and sizes of people. For example, very large, heavy individuals require firmer, more supportive bedding. A mattress that is too firm, however, can also cause stress for some body types. For example, obese people who sleep on extra-firm bedding may experience pooling of body fluids, oxygen deprivation, tissue stagnation, and inflammation. These effects can cause symptoms such as morning stiffness and an assortment of aches and pains, especially in the elbows, hips, knee joints, and shoulders. This isn't true only for people with obesity, however. Very thin people who have little protective fat may also experience joint pain and stiffness. Every doctor has treated patients with painful, even temporarily disabling, bursitis of the elbows, hips, or shoulders—all symptoms experienced by either very heavy or very thin people using mattresses and bedding that are too firm. One way to ensure that you benefit from a balance of firmness and cushioning if you have a firm or extra-firm mattress is to purchase a one- or two-inch thick piece of soft foam cushion, available at your local fabric or upholstery store. Put the foam cushion on top of your mattress and secure it with a traditional mattress cover. Another option is to purchase a goose-down-filled cushion that can be placed over your mattress. You should be able to find such cushions in the bedding section of department stores or in specialty catalogues that feature such items.

Water Beds, Air Beds, and Conventional Bedding

Many patients ask whether waterbeds or inflatable airbeds are preferred over traditional coiled-spring mattresses. While this varies from person to person, people with a medium-range body mass—neither very large and heavy nor unusually thin—have more options when choosing bedding. As a general rule, it's always a good idea to purchase bedding from a retailer who is knowledgeable about the benefits of different bedding for different body types. If you are considering purchasing a water or air mattress, it's best to speak to a dealer who sells these types of mattresses as well as conventional bedding because they will generally be more candid about the best features of all of these choices. If your sleeping partner is significantly heavier or lighter than you are, it may be best to purchase bedding that can be adjusted on either side of the bed to accommodate each of your unique needs. Air beds that have individual adjustable chambers for each side of the bed can be very helpful in these cases.

Some of the name-brand mattress companies I have recommended over the years are Serta, Simmons, and Springwall. In addition, some of my patients have also reported positive benefits from a new bedding concept featuring a foam material sensitive to body heat that conforms to different body shapes and sizes. The Tempur-Pedic Pressure-Relieving Swedish Mattress and Pillow system is the only mattress recognized by NASA and certified by the Space Foundation. The company also manufactures a variety of other neck and back support products that are available in specialty stores in malls and shopping centers. For further information, consult their website at www.tempurpedic.com.

Pillows

As important as choosing the proper mattress is selecting just the right pillow. Many people can benefit from a specially designed contour pillow that has a recess for the head and support for the neck. My personal choices are the temperature-sensitive Tempur-Pedic pillow that uses body heat to mold to the shape of your neck, and the P.F. Pillow. The P.F. pillow contains sterilized premium white goose down and is fitted with a medium-density foam cervical support that is sewn into the fabric. The foam insert is tapered for optimal comfort and provides excellent support for the neck. For further information, consult their website at www.PFPillows.com.

If you have wide shoulders and are most comfortable sleeping on your side, you will probably need a thicker than average pillow to keep your neck and head in alignment with the rest your spine. On the other hand, if you have a small frame and narrow shoulders, or prefer to sleep mainly on your back, you may wish to choose a thinner pillow to keep your body comfortably aligned.

Electric Blankets

I do not recommend using electric blankets. The human body is itself an electrical energy system that operates on a 60-cycle direct current, whereas electric blankets operate on the traditional 110-volt alternating current. Surrounding yourself in an electrical field that is not compatible with the body's natural energy cycle can be harmful.

SLEEP POSTURES

Avoid sleeping on your abdomen. It twists the neck, distorts the pelvis, and results in excessive strain on the joints, muscles, and nerves of your neck and lower spine. Sleeping on your back is acceptable, provided you are using a properly shaped and supportive pillow for your neck. For most people, however, side sleeping is best, with your knees moderately flexed to reduce the strain of your lower spinal muscles. Placing your hand or arm beneath your head and face while sleeping is not a good idea. This indicates a need for a thicker pillow, because you're using your hand or arm to add support for the head and neck to keep the spine in proper alignment. In general, it's best to keep your arms below your shoulders when sleeping.

INSOMNIA

Insomnia can be a challenging health concern, and many physical and emotional factors can play a role in both its cause and its cure. Physically, for example, insomnia is often the result of a magnesium deficiency. Most adults need 400–800 mg of magnesium a day, yet up to 80 percent of Americans have mild, moderate, or severe magnesium deficiency. When combined with calcium and vitamins C and D, magnesium can benefit your sleep and your overall health. Isn't it remarkable that taking such a simple and safe step can be so effective—and can literally change your life? With these thoughts in mind, if you suffer from insomnia, you may first wish to address the sources of physical or psychological stress in your life before you resort to sleeping pills. In addition, follow this time-honored, commonsense advice for a good night's sleep:

- Avoid caffeine or other stimulating chemicals, particularly after noon. These stimulants include coffee, black and green teas, most soft drinks, chocolate, and various over-the-counter pain and allergy medications.

- Do not eat a large dinner just prior to bedtime.

- Drink relaxing herbal teas before bed, such as chamomile or Sleepy Time.

- Use valerian root, a safe, effective herbal supplement that facilitates sleep (as needed).

- Maintain a consistent bedtime.

- Use comfortable, supportive bedding.

- Choose the right size, shape, and texture pillow for your comfort.

- Use adequate covering for warmth.

- Keep your bedroom at a comfortable temperature.

- Make sure your windows are adequately shaded for near-total darkness.

- Maintain a peaceful, quiet, and relaxing atmosphere.

- Wear comfortable, nonconstrictive sleepwear.

- Avoid watching sensational and violent television before bedtime.

- Don't *try* to fall asleep.

If you share a bed with another person, it's important that she or he respects your sleep requirements and takes steps to help the process. For example, a bed partner who consistently snores loudly can be a very serious deterrent to sound sleep. If you or your sleep partner snores, try using the Breathe Rite adhesive strips available at any drug store. Since snoring is usually a result of sleeping on the back, and because sleep-posture habits are unconscious, you may have to gently nudge your partner, and ask him or her to shift to either side. If your partner finds it difficult to overcome the habit of sleeping on his or her back, it may be helpful to tape a golf or tennis ball to your partner's back shortly before turning the lights out and going to sleep. A week or two of this tactic should help reprogram sleep posture. If you are not able to find a solution for snoring, it may be necessary for you and your partner to sleep in separate beds, or even separate bedrooms, to assure adequate sleep. Keep in mind, your health depends significantly on adequate rest and sleep. It's imperative for you and your partner to honor each other's needs in this regard. This simple courtesy can greatly benefit long-term love relationships.

To facilitate drowsiness as you lie there wide awake, try to actually count sheep. Or anything else you'd prefer to count for that matter. For example, if you have a large extended family—as I do—try counting your cousins. You might even try counting your blessings, and may be amazed at how richly your life has been blessed. While something so simple may sound like an old wives' tale, this technique can actually help you fall asleep if it shifts your focus from the stress of your worries and fears to more positive thoughts.

What measures should you take if you have tried all of the above common-sense approaches to natural sleep, and you continue to suffer from insomnia? Before you reach for the sleeping pills, you may wish to consider the use of melatonin supplements. Melatonin is a naturally occurring hormone secreted by the pineal gland that helps regulate the body's natural circadian rhythm and sleep cycles. It is available without prescription and has been valuable for certain individuals who struggle with insomnia. Since melatonin can affect the body's hormonal system, it may be wise to speak to your doctor or pharmacist about whether it is appropriate for your particular needs before using it for an extended period.

REM SLEEP AND DEEP SLEEP

Others can tell when you are dreaming because your eyeballs actively move behind your eyelids as if your eyes were consciously seeing or observing a scene. This is known as REM (rapid eye movement) sleep. REM sleep monitored electronically with instruments that measure brain-wave activity has shown that, during the dream phase, brain wave activity is similar to when we are consciously awake.

Deep sleep is another phase of sleep that we all experience. During deep sleep, it is unlikely that you dream, because the brain is much less active. Various studies have shown that REM sleep and deep sleep are equally important body functions, and being deprived of either or both can have numerous negative effects on your health and efficient function.

So what purpose do our dreams serve? When we dream, the neurons in the brain unscramble their circuitry while they are not being used for thinking and reasoning. These dreams are almost never remembered. On the other hand, if you experience emotionally disturbing dreams, or nightmares that you readily recall upon awakening and that remain on your mind the next day, your dream state could be attempting to convey information to you. This is especially true if you have the same nightmare over and over. If this is the case, you should try to figure out the deeper meaning of the dream and even ask a professional to help you interpret your recurrent dreams, if necessary.

Dreams

Did you know that dreaming is valuable to your mental, physical, and spiritual well-being, and is, therefore, important to your health? In our culture, however, dreams are generally thought to have little or no significance. Most investigators stress the physical effects of REM sleep deprivation, putting little emphasis on dreams themselves. By contrast, holistically oriented practitioners place an emphasis on the emotional and spiritual aspects of dreams, and believe we can benefit from a better understanding of their significance in maintaining health. In my professional experience, I have found that most people take their dreams completely for granted, pay almost no attention to them, or say they do not remember them. When recalling their dreams, they either find humor in them, or feel that the dreams are so unstructured, they have no value or meaning. While it's true that most of our dreams are likely to have little or no importance to our conscious experience, it's well known that every person dreams at least several hours during each sleep cycle. This may come as a surprise, particularly if you do not remember your dreams. But rest assured, the mind *does* engage in the dream process even if you don't recall your dreams the next day. And, this being the case, it only makes sense to consider dreams an important aspect of the human experience, and to recognize that learning more about this area of your existence could be helpful to you.

Interpreting Dreams

The following story will illustrate the role that interpreting a recurring nightmare played in the care of one of my seriously ill patients.

Louise had been referred to me for arthritis and the degeneration in her spine, hips, knees, and ankles that had become progressively more disabling every year. She moved very slowly and was in obvious pain as she entered my consultation room. Using two sturdy wooden canes to help support her every step, this large-boned, significantly overweight woman could barely fit between the armrests of the generously sized chair next to my desk. In reviewing the comprehensive history form Louise had filled out, I noted she wrote that, in addition to having advanced stages of osteoarthritis and osteoporosis for many years, she also had bloating, congestive heart failure, extreme fatigue, fluid retention, high blood pressure, long-standing constipation, and shortness of breath. She listed ten separate prescription drugs that she took, along with several over-the-counter pain relievers. Louise said she almost never drank water, but did drink about ten cups of coffee a day and two or three cans of diet soda. She needed the caffeine, she said, to help her stay awake because she was always tired. She simply was not getting enough sleep due to the same recurring nightmare, a nightmare that she had experienced many times over a forty-year span.

After a series of careful evaluations, our discussion centered on a program that would include natural, non-drug approaches to try and provide her with some relief from her severely disabling symptoms. Because virtually all the joints of her lower extremities, as well as her spine, were almost totally degenerated, I had to explain to her it was unlikely we would be able to provide substantial relief. Having been to many other doctors, and having tried many drugs and other forms of treatment, she understood the challenges facing her. However, I informed her that if she was willing to faithfully follow my advice, there could be some hope for improvement.

In just a few office visits, I sensed that Louise had developed a greater level of trust and confidence in me, so I inquired about her sleep difficulties and the recurrent nightmares that woke her. She was very embarrassed about the horrible recurring dream she had, and told me it was awful to describe—so disgusting, in fact, that she had never revealed it to anyone, not even her husband, who had unsuccessfully tried to get her to a psychiatrist. I assured her any information she chose to share with me would be totally confidential, and I went on to explain that recurring dreams sometimes contain important information that affects health. After several successful treatment sessions, she decided to open up on this very sensitive topic, and she told me about the nightmare. I have paraphrased it below using the first person.

> "I dream I am alone in a big, old house. In the early years of the dream, I am sitting on the second floor bathroom commode, but when I am finished using it, the toilet does not flush. For several years, the dream stayed essentially the same, but gradually it started to change—not only wouldn't the toilet flush, the waste would spill over the edge of the stool and create a foul mess in the bathroom. As years passed, the dream became increasingly more frequent, and more and more realistic and disgusting, with the waste not only engulfing the entire bathroom, but also the upstairs bedrooms. After a while, the waste was contaminating the entire first floor of the house as well. It is always just awful and I wake up in a state of panic and am afraid to fall back to sleep. For the past ten years or so, the theme of the dream has been the same, it just comes more frequently, and every year there is more and more destruction in the house because of the overflowing toilet. In recent years, the entire basement and the foundation of the house are also crumbling. Just before I wake up, I feel the whole house crashing down on top of me and I wake up screaming."

When she finished, she was weeping silently and was obviously relieved to finally be confiding in someone about this terrible recurring nightmare that had been troubling her for over forty years. I reassured her that while some dreams may have literal meanings, most are symbolic, and I explained the basic symbols that were emerging in her nightmare. I suggested that she might interpret the big, old house as her body, and the walls and foundation of the house as her skeleton. The body is also the home of the soul—it's where the soul "lives." Just as the house itself is symbolic, each room in the house also has a symbolic meaning. For example, the kitchen may represent your cooking habits, while the dining room signifies your eating habits. Along these lines, the living room or family room may symbolize your family life, while the music room or library could be representative of artistic or intellectual pursuits, and the bedroom is usually symbolic of sleep habits or sexual activities. Following this line of reasoning, the bathroom represents cleansing the body. In greater detail, a shower or bath suggests washing your skin and hair, whereas using the toilet is symbolic of cleansing your inner organs and eliminating toxic wastes from your body.

As I explained the symbolic meaning of the dream to Louise, her eyes widened and she began to weep again, this time from a sense of understanding. "Yes, that's it. I finally understand," she said. What she finally understood was that her psyche, or higher-consciousness was warning her, through her dream state, about the bad habits and the chronic constipation she had struggled with since her teenage years, and the health-robbing toxicity that had resulted. Although it was unfortunately too late to make major, lasting changes in her health, from that point on she never again experienced the recurring nightmare, and she was finally able to sleep through the night.

I hope Louise's story helps you understand how some of your worst nightmares can be your most helpful and valuable dreams. Each dream is a gift. Learn to nurture, welcome, and cherish your dreams, including—and especially—your bad dreams. Some consider them the way to have a meaningful dialog with your higher self. While the interpretation of most dreams may not be as obvious as in the story of Louise, it is important to place this aspect of our lives in proper perspective. Our dreams usually incorporate visual images, colors, sounds, aromas, emotions, numbers, people, and other symbols to convey their message. Since the majority of dreams are simple, you can look to the obvious meanings most of the time. Try keeping a dream journal to regularly jot down the dreams you most vividly recall. This is a way to find similar dream patterns or themes emerging, so you don't have to evaluate each dream separately. Over time, you may come to realize that your dreams can be trustworthy, helpful guides for your physical, emotional, and spiritual well-being.

If you would like to learn more about the basic principles of assessing and analyzing your dreams, there are many worthwhile books and scientific articles on the topic. My all-time favorite dream book is *Dreams, Your Magic Mirror* by Elsie Sechrist. Another highly recommended book about dreams is *The Secret Language of Dreams: A Visual Key to Dreams and their Meanings* by Dr. David Fontana. For further information on dreams, as well as in-depth information on sleep, insomnia, and sleep disorders, contact the American Academy of Sleep Medicine at 708-492-0930 or www.aasmnet.org.

8. Fresh Air and Breathing

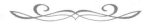

his vital Golden Rule relates to the importance of the air you breathe, and to obtaining adequate oxygen. While you can live for approximately three weeks without food and about three days without water, you can survive only a few minutes without air and the critical element it provides—oxygen. The importance of taking in enough oxygen cannot be overemphasized. Equally important is the process of expelling carbon dioxide and other waste products from the bloodstream, which is also a function of breathing.

PROPER BREATHING TECHNIQUE

You may not realize that for optimal health and energy, it's important to breathe properly. Most people, particularly women, breathe with only the upper third of their lungs. This shallow breathing starves the blood of oxygen and causes an excess of waste products to accumulate in the body. To avoid these negative health effects, you should develop the habit of breathing deeply from your diaphragm and abdomen, inhaling deeply through your nose, and slowly blowing the air out from deep in your abdomen and diaphragm through pursed lips. The diaphragm is a dome-shaped, crisscrossing layered muscle that separates the chest cavity from the abdominal cavity. It's a powerful muscle that acts as a bellows to move air in and out of your lungs when you breathe. Breathing in deeply is important, of course, but breathing out is equally important because that's how the body rids itself of carbon dioxide and other waste products to keep rich, oxygen-filled red blood cells flowing through the bloodstream. The diaphragm also plays an important role in heart function by acting as another pump to return venous blood back to the heart from the lower extremities, which helps your general circulation.

Another simple yet effective breathing exercise is to blow air out through a straw, using muscles from deep in your abdomen. It's also very important to develop the habit of breathing through your nose, as this allows the sinus cavities to warm and filter the air before it enters your lungs. Practice these techniques as often as you can, particularly when you feel stress accumulating. For example, deep-breathing exercises can help you relax in the car commuting to and from work—although it's probably not a good idea to do so while you are waiting at the light, or locked in a traffic jam because of the high levels of carbon monoxide. However, be aware that some powerful deep-breathing exercises can make you feel lightheaded, so stop immediately if that is the case because you certainly don't want to black out while driving.

Breathing and Posture

Poor breathing results in poor posture and proper breathing results in improved posture, so deep, full-body breathing is a great way to improve your posture. The way you carry yourself, move your body through space, and maintain your posture are some of the most significant features of your attractiveness and confidence, and an expression of vibrant good health.

To function efficiently, the muscles required to maintain good posture need substantial amounts of oxygen, which they take in from the air you breathe. These muscles also obtain essential nutrients from food through the arterial blood—nutrients that are required to maintain their normal muscle tone, strength, and excitability. When you slouch and breathe only from the upper third of your lungs, your muscles are deprived of vital oxygen and nutrients, and this results in muscle fatigue and poor circulation.

The diaphragm helps maintain good posture because it attaches to the spinal column in back and the rib cage in front. Shallow breathers have a sunken-chest appearance, whereas people who breathe deeply from the abdomen carry themselves tall and give off an appearance of confidence, vitality, and youth.

AIR QUANTITY AND QUALITY

It is well known that the oxygen content of the air we breathe has been gradually decreasing since the advent of the industrial revolution in the nineteenth century, primarily as a result of burning fossil fuels in motorized vehicles, and industrial factories, as well as deforestation. The exact effect of this on human health remains unknown, but common sense dictates that continuously breathing contaminated air has to have negative effects on your health. Airborne contaminants can be either organic—pollens, molds, wood dust, agricultural dusts from the manure of hogs or poultry, and molds from grains or hay—or inorganic particles associated with building, mining, and road construction. For example, if you live in a large city, you are most likely breathing in polluted air, including varying amounts of carbon monoxide, asbestos, benzene, car exhaust, diesel smoke, lead, and micro-particles of rubber tires. Also, depending on the city and the prevailing winds, airborne industrial and chemical contaminants of varying quantity and toxicity may also be circulating in your air supply. Many of these contaminants are absorbed into the bloodstream, posing a threat to your immune system and the rest of your body functions.

Diseases such as asbestosis, emphysema, silicosis, and a wide variety of less serious illnesses can all result from the air you are breathing. Many times these respiratory illnesses are difficult to detect because they can take several years to manifest, yet their effects can be permanent, irreversible, and even fatal. This is particularly true if you are a smoker, or if you unintentionally inhale significant amounts of secondhand smoke.

Did you know that in the United States eight coal miners die every day as the result of black lung disease? But it's not just construction workers, miners, and people working in grain elevators who are at risk for air contamination. After a distance runner completes a twenty-six-mile race—the Boston Marathon, for example—he or she will have inhaled an amount of carbon monoxide equivalent to smoking three packs of cigarettes. This might make you wonder about the supposed health and fitness benefits for a long-distance runner, particularly if most of the training and participation takes place in a large urban area.

Sick-Building Syndrome

By now, most people are aware of the possibility of chemical and toxic exposure in their work environments. This awareness is due in large part to the publicity generated by the case in which a number of hotel guests attending an American Legion Convention who suddenly died from a condition later called Legionnaire's Disease. After much investigation, it was discovered that the illness was the result of microbes in the building's air ducts. Health risks such as this and others in large air-conditioned buildings are real, and if you believe your health is being affected by such factors at work, you owe it to yourself and to your co-workers to help your employer track down the source of contamination and minimize the risk. Employers who become aware of airborne contamination in the workplace often hire professionally trained industrial hygienists to identify the problem and correct it.

Sick-Building Syndrome in the Home

When you consider that there are 168 hours in a week, and that the average person spends less than one-fourth of his or her time in the workplace, it may also be important to consider the notion of sick-building syndrome in your own home. It's currently estimated that as many as 10 million Americans have multiple chemical sensitivities (MCS), a condition also known as environmental illness, that is often associated with chronic fatigue syndrome and fibromyalgia. The home can be a primary source of these illnesses.

While you would expect our healthcare system to be well-aware of the symptoms of MCS, people with this condition usually have to go from doctor to doctor, specialist to specialist, and literally struggle for years before their condition is recognized and treated. Why is the condition so difficult to diagnose? For one reason, the onset of symptoms is gradual, including aches and pains, airway obstruction, fatigue, flu-like symptoms, headaches, nausea, skin rashes, and wheezing. Furthermore, in most cases the person is not acutely ill, and most traditional and comprehensive medical examinations reveal few positive findings.

In cases of MCS, the culprits are often seemingly innocuous factors, such as newly installed carpeting, kitchen cabinets, insulation, or paneling, all of which can release large amounts of formaldehyde and trigger a severe reaction in people who are environmentally sensitive to the chemical. Household cleaning products—including aerosol sprays, air fresheners, cleansers, disinfectants, paints, and solvents—are often sources of toxic or carcinogenic (cancer-causing) substances that may contribute to MCS. Fireplaces, gas ranges, and water heaters can release small amounts of carbon monoxide, and some people are sensitive to the chemical added to natural gas, which normally has no odor, to warn of gas leaks. Mildew and molds from wet or damp basements, and poorly maintained air conditioners and humidifiers can often cause or aggravate the condition, as can the chemicals used in dry-cleaning. And obviously, herbicides, insecticides, lawn fertilizers, and rodent controls are on the list of items to avoid.

What Can You Do About MCS?

If you don't think you are affected by MCS, it is important to realize that the condition is often misdiagnosed as something else. Whether you already struggle with environmental illnesses, or you're looking to reduce your risk, conduct a careful evaluation of your home to ascertain possible sources of chemical hazards.

To reduce contaminants—including airborne contaminants—in your environment, consider using electric stoves, furnaces, and water heaters, rather than gas-powered appliances. Use nontoxic household cleaning products. If you are making improvements to your home, choose only solid wood cabinets and furniture rather than products made from potentially toxic particleboard and glues. If you have known sensitivities, you may need to avoid carpeted floors, choosing instead wood, ceramic, stone, tile, or other durable, non-porous materials. Carefully maintain humidifiers, dehumidifiers, and air conditioners, and make absolutely certain that your ventilation system brings in sufficient amounts of outside air, especially during winter months. Use fans to circulate fresh air and remove stale or contaminated air, often generated by stoves and indoor barbecue systems. Use nontoxic pest, rodent, and weed-control methods. Have your general water supply—used for bathing, cleaning, and cooking—tested for arsenic, lead, mercury, or other contamination, and filter your drinking water.

Filter Your Air

To eliminate common airborne contaminants, such as dusts, mildew, and molds, you may wish to consider investing in a high-quality air-filtering system This is especially important for people with chronic respiratory or allergic conditions, including asthma, emphysema, hay fever, MCS, or sinusitis.

A wide selection of air purifiers and air filtration systems are available, including models manufactured by Amway (E-2526), Honeywell (13520 HEPA), Shaklee (Air Source), Sharper Image (Quadra B), and Whirlpool (450). Features and prices of each vary greatly. When purchasing an air purifier or filter, consider the space in which you will put it to use, because some appliances are designed for small spaces, such as individual bedrooms or offices, while others are designed to filter the air of an average-size home. Carefully review and compare the performance features, costs, upkeep, and energy requirements before making your purchase. To determine the role of air filtration in reducing your allergies, visit www.Allernet.com.

Should You Consider Using an Ozone Generator?

While ozone is a necessary part of the upper atmosphere, it's also a principle component of smog in the lower atmosphere, including the air we breathe in large cities—and it's a potent lung irritant that can cause respiratory distress. Ozone is a powerful oxidizing agent, and the levels of the element that clean air effectively are unsafe for human health. Long-term exposure to high levels of ozone can result in permanent lung damage; cough and chest pain during deep inhalation; eye, nose, and throat irritation; and increased sensitivity to airborne allergens and irritants. Additionally, ozone can react with volatile compounds in the air to produce harmful byproducts such as formaldehyde. Children, older people, and individuals with respiratory diseases such as asthma are most susceptible to the toxic effects of ozone.

There is some debate surrounding the use of home or office ozone generators, which are often marketed in conjunction with home air-filtration systems. The American Lung Association recommends that people who are seeking cleaner indoor air avoid the use of ozone-generating devices for the reasons discussed above. Consumers who are interested in buying an electronic air cleaner would be wise to research which filtration systems have been tested for ozone production. Filters or electrostatic precipitators may be safer methods of cleaning indoor air, and may be more effective than devices that generate ozone.

The U.S. Food and Drug Administration prohibits the sale of devices that include more than fifty parts of ozone per billion in the air of occupied, enclosed spaces, such as homes, offices, or vehicles. The levels of ozone generated by a device are influenced by many factors, such as the power setting, the room size, and the ventilation rate, and therefore are not easily controlled by the consumer.

Restore Your Health—Restore the Health of Your Home

Given the above information, you can readily understand the potential health risks of simply living in your house. Sick-building syndrome is more than a metaphor, and the sickest building may be the one in which you probably spend most of your time—your home. You can read more on this important topic in Richard Leviton's excellent book *The Healthy Living Space,* which expands on many issues that could be important to preserving or restoring your health.

Electro-Dermal Screening (EDS) Can Help

If you know or suspect that you suffer from chemical sensitivities, electro-dermal screening (EDS) can be very helpful in your efforts to minimize and eliminate the exposure factors. EDS testing is an inexpensive yet efficient way for a healthcare professional to evaluate your sensitivity to thousands of potentially harmful environmental agents, and homeopathic remedies can often dramatically assist in your recovery. (See Chapter 9 for a more in-depth description of EDS.) For a list of doctors and clinics that provide electro-dermal screening, contact NuHealth Wellness at their website www.nuhealthwellness.com.

ADDITIONAL RESOURCES

If you feel you may have multiple chemical sensitivities (MCS) or environmental illness, and your efforts have failed to bring you relief, any of the following organizations may provide the help you need:

American Academy of Environmental Medicine: www.aaem.com

American Academy of Otolaryngic Allergy: www.allergy-ENT.com

American Chemical Society: www.acs.org

The Healthy House Institute: www.hhinst.com

Multiple Chemical Sensitivity Referral and Resources: www.mcsrr.org

9. Choosing Your Doctors and Care Providers

Even if you are healthy, it's essential to have access to healthcare providers, and you should be selective when choosing them. The difference in the skills, experience, and attitudes of healthcare professionals could either save or threaten your life. This Golden Rule focuses on the next area of importance in preserving your health: the selection of healthcare professionals when you need them.

HOLISTIC HEALTH CARE

When possible, try to find holistically oriented physicians, nurses, and other healthcare professionals who believe that the body is more than the sum of its parts. These practitioners embrace the notion that all living species, including humans, possess innate intelligence that serves to maintain the body's health and integrity, and that the role of the doctor or health practitioner is to facilitate and enhance this response.

Ideally, any healthcare provider you choose should also subscribe to the following practices and beliefs:

- Optimal health is a manifestation of harmony within the body, mind, and spirit.

- A healthcare professional should be knowledgeable about, and supportive of, all forms of healing, and must be familiar with various approaches to health care in order to present patients with the most effective, safest preventive or treatment options available.

- A care provider should emphasize prevention and whole-person wellness, and teach healthy living practices.

- The care-provider/patient relationship is one of mutual respect.

- Other than for acute, potentially life-threatening emergencies, the patient should be involved in decisions regarding his or her own medical care. In instances where the patient's condition or age prevents active participation in his or her own health care—infants, children, and adults who are significantly dependent on others, for example—family members are involved in these decisions.

- The patient's attitudes, beliefs, and interpersonal relationships are considered important contributors to health and well-being.

- The patient's relationship with all of nature and the physical environment of the earth are important in the holistic model of health care.

- The patient is primarily responsible for his or her own health.

This holistic model of health care is one we should all envision for the future. It empowers and enables us to move from being passive recipients to active participants in attaining and maintaining health by embracing the concepts of self-responsibility and informed choice. The late Dr. Keith Sehnert is considered one of the pioneers in patient empowerment and the holistic healthcare movement in this country. His book *How to Be Your Own Doctor—Sometimes* is well worth reading.

ALTERNATIVE AND COMPLEMENTARY FORMS OF HEALING

An increased volume of factual evidence has demonstrated the value of alternative and complementary forms of healing, and it is important to remain open-minded and willing to explore these various options. Acupuncture, aromatherapy, Ayurvedic healing, Chinese medicine, chiropractic, creative visualization, herbal and botanical medicine, homeopathy, massage, myofascial release therapy, naturopathy, qigong, Reiki, and other alternative forms of health care are gaining in stature and respectability, and are becoming more widely available. Many of these forms of health care are regulated by licenses and require extensive training and clinical experience. Because some forms of care may be more effective than others in meeting your unique needs, ask friends and family members for referrals to providers who may be helpful for your particular condition. In addition, holistically oriented doctors of all disciplines often provide referrals to other practitioners who provide services they are not trained to offer and who may be greatly beneficial to you.

Acupuncture

Acupuncture is a system of healing that has been a major component of traditional Chinese medicine for over 3,000 years. It is based on the belief that optimal health is achieved by maintaining the flow and balance of life energy throughout the body. In Eastern medicine, this energy is called ch'i—often spelled qi and pronounced *chee* in Chinese and *kee* in Japanese—and it is divided into two polarities known as yin and yang. Ch'i energy flows through the body along energy pathways known as *meridians,* with each meridian's name based on the organ or system with which it corresponds. Twelve of the meridians are the bladder; gallbladder; heart; kidney; large intestine; liver; lung; pericardium, which controls circulation; small intestine; spleen and pancreas; stomach; and triple heater, which controls the glandular system of the body. Two additional pathways, the conception and governor meridians, travel up and down the midline of the body and overlap the circulatory and nervous systems, but also remain separate from them. Many believe that the energy flow of acupuncture meridians fluctuates with the body's electromagnetic field, and for that reason, acupuncture is referred to as a form of energy medicine.

Acupuncture meridians are stimulated or sedated by inserting tiny stainless steel needles at specific acupuncture points located on the skin. The specific points chosen by the clinician depend on whether there is an excess or a deficiency of ch'i present in that meridian. Yin is considered passive, contracting, and cold, whereas its balancing energy polarity, yang, is active, external, and warm. If there is an excess of yin energy, it automatically creates a deficiency of yang energy and vice versa. Acupuncture theory maintains that, uncorrected, the imbalance will lead to sickness or dysfunction. Acupuncture points are also referred to as gates, and master acupuncturists have identified as many as 2,000 acupuncture points that can influence yin/yang balance within the meridians. Meridian imbalance is determined by evidence of a disturbance in various body functions. Included in traditional Chinese medicine are subtle systems known as pulse and tongue diagnoses that also help the practitioner identify energy imbalances in the body. Other means of affecting acupuncture points include acupressure, which is manual contact with acupuncture points, moxibustion, a form of local heat application, in concert with the acupuncture needles; and laser energy.

Millions worldwide have experienced the many benefits of acupuncture diagnosis and treatment. Some of the documented outcomes of successful acupuncture treatment include an enhanced immune system function; headache relief, including migraines; improved function of the female reproductive system; improved heart, respiratory, and circulatory functions; improved digestive function; and smoking cessation. It is also very popular in treating musculoskeletal pain. In Eastern medicine, acupuncture is used as anesthesia for various surgical and dental procedures. Traditional acupuncturists place great emphasis on lifestyle, nutrition, exercise, fresh air, rest, and sleep.

Aromatherapy

The practice of aromatherapy uses essential oils extracted from selected plants for therapeutic purposes, a technique that dates back to ancient times. In Eastern and Middle-Eastern countries, oils were used initially only as perfumes, but ancient physicians began to find value for these therapeutic oils for massages and in healing baths, and gradually extended their applications to treat a wide variety of diseases. Over the ages, a refinement of distillation processes and application techniques has restored aromatherapy to a respected position in the healing arts, and many people now use essential oils to help achieve better emotional and physical health, as aromatic oils have both a physical effect and a psychological value in the healing process. The oils are absorbed through the pores of the skin and the lining of the respiratory and digestive systems to affect all the organs and systems of the body.

Essential oils are extracted from the bark, flowers, leaves, roots, and seeds of whole bushes, herbs, shrubs, and trees, and must be 100 percent pure for healing purposes. There are a variety of ways to use these oils, including air diffusion, baths, compresses, inhalation, and massage, and they can even be added, in very small doses, to honey, soups, sugar, teas, or water.

The most commonly used aromatherapy oils are chamomile, clary, sage, eucalyptus, jasmine, lavender, lemon, oregano, peppermint, rosemary, sandalwood, and tea tree oils. Aromatherapy can be incorporated into the treatment of a wide variety of problems and conditions, including anxiety, arthritis, bladder infections, burns, circulation problems, depression, headaches, indigestion, insomnia, menstrual pains, muscular aches and pains, respiratory disorders, and skin conditions.

It's important to clearly understand the safest way to use essential oils. For example, some full-strength oils can be irritating to the skin, eyes, and mucous membranes, and are meant to be diluted and used only where applicable. To learn more about this fascinating healing system, I recommend reading *The Practice of Aromatherapy* by Jean Valnet, M.D.

Ayurvedic Medicine

The term Ayurveda is from the Sanskrit words *ayur* (life) and *veda* (knowledge or science). Ayurvedic medicine is the traditional healing system of India and traces its history to ancient Hindu teachings and texts. Similar to other ancient health practices, Ayurveda is a natural, holistic approach to healing that emphasizes preventing illness, rather than waiting until an illness occurs to seek treatment. In Ayurvedic philosophy, health is the result of life-giving energies flowing through all the various organs and systems of the body, and illness is an expression of imbalance in these energies. Thus, treatment is aimed at restoring energy balances throughout the body, and may include dietary advice, enemas, fasting, herbal preparations, homeopathic medicines, inhalations, massages, nutritional supplementation, special baths, and exposure to sunshine. Yoga, meditation, and special breathing techniques are other aspects of Ayurvedic medicine that are considered important to both physical and emotional well-being. To better acquaint yourself with the theories and applications of Ayurvedic medicine, I encourage you to read Dr. Deepak Chopra's *Perfect Health—The Complete Mind/Body Guide.*

Traditional Chinese Medicine

The history of traditional Chinese internal medicine, or Chinese herbalism, can be traced back 5,000 years or more. Current Chinese herbal medicine practices are based largely on a book written around 200 B.C. known as the *Huang Ti Nei-Ching (Yellow Emperor's Manual of Internal Medicine),* in which herbs and herbal combinations are the principle healing agents discussed. Through the years, there has been a gradual, steady increase in the number of healing herbs used in this ancient system of holistic health care, and today, over 5,000 herbal remedies are regularly used in China and other countries. Chinese herbal medicine is rapidly gaining popularity in the United States.

Traditional Chinese medicine is based on the Taoist philosophy that emphasizes the importance of balance and unimpeded flow of life forces in the body known as ch'i or qi. As previously discussed, the ch'i energy flows are composed of yin and yang, which are opposite polarities counterbalancing each other. Illness or disease results from an imbalance of yin and yang due to blockages or deficiencies in the flow of these life-force energies. Carefully harvested and selected Chinese herbal remedies are used to restore energy, balance, and harmony in order to treat a wide variety of physical, mental, and emotional conditions, including chronic conditions such as arthritis; chronic fatigue syndrome;

digestive, reproductive, and respiratory system disorders; migraine headaches; and skin conditions.

Because herbs and herbal combinations represent sophisticated biochemistry, people with serious health problems, particularly those using one or more conventional medications, should be aware of herb/drug interactions that could cause disturbing and even dangerous side effects. Women who are pregnant or breastfeeding should use medications, including herbal preparations, only with the advice and supervision of a health-care practitioner. *The Web That Has No Weaver* by Ted Kapchuk and *Between Heaven and Earth* by Bienfeld and Kornbloom are two references books I recommend to build your understanding of Chinese herbal medicine.

Chiropractic

Chiropractic was founded in 1895 by natural healer, David Daniel Palmer. The word chiropractic is derived from the Greek *cheiro* (hand) and *praktikos* (to do). From this, you can surmise that chiropractic places significant emphasis on manual means of evaluating and treating the body. At the present time, there are licensed chiropractors in every state in the United States and in over one hundred countries and about 94 percent of all skilled manipulative care in the world is provided by doctors of chiropractic. With approximately 67,000 practicing doctors, chiropractic is the second largest primary healthcare system in the United States, after M.D.s, and there are another 20,000 chiropractors in other countries.

As a holistic, drugless, non-surgical system of healing, chiropractic is based on the premise that inborn wisdom exists in all living organisms, including humans, and regulates all the body's glands, internal organs, and systems. In chiropractic circles, this wisdom is known as innate intelligence, and the concept is similar to the Latin phrase *viz mediacatrix naturae,* the healing power of nature, expressed by holistically oriented physicians who practice Western medicine. This self-regulating, self-healing power is the life force that regulates homeostasis, the natural harmony or balance within the body.

Chiropractic draws on the theory that the nervous system—consisting of the brain, spinal cord, cranial and spinal nerves, autonomic nervous system, and special sense organs, such as the eyes and ears—controls all of the body's other organs and structures and relates the body to its environment to maintain homeostasis. According to chiropractic philosophy, there is an intimate relationship between structure and function, and the integrity of the body's structure must be maintained in order to preserve optimal function. Its major premise is that impairments to the body's framework, especially in the spine, can cause disturbances in the nervous system, thus affecting nerve energy, or innate intelligence. This interrelating disturbance is known as the subluxation complex. Subluxation refers to an existing disturbance in one or more of the joints of the body, but particularly in the spine, that can interfere with the function of the nervous system.

Chiropractors are skilled in the detection and reduction of the subluxation complex through carefully determined, and specifically directed, manual or mechanical corrective procedures known as chiropractic adjustments. Prior to making the adjustment, the chiropractor performs a wide range of clinical diagnostic and evaluation procedures, including a thorough medical history, a traditional physical examination, a postural and biomechanical assessment, muscle testing, chemical laboratory analysis, x-rays, and other specialized evaluations, as needed. Most chiropractors also provide soft-tissue manipulation, as well as a variety of physical therapies such as heat, cold, light, ultrasound, and electricity. Significant emphasis is also placed on exercise, lifestyle, nutrition, occupational and sports-related concerns, physical fitness, stress management, and stretching.

People who can greatly benefit from chiropractic care are those who are experiencing neuromusculoskeletal disorders, particularly work-related and athletic injuries, including arthritis, back, neck, and extremity pain, repetitive strain, sciatica, or whiplash. Additionally, chiropractic can be helpful in managing headaches, including migraines. Perhaps more surprising, however, is the fact that recent research has documented chiropractic's efficacy in treating conditions such as asthma, digestive disorders, menstrual problems, and other health disturbances resulting from the subluxation complex.

A great variety of chiropractic techniques are offered by chiropractors, and each has its own unique value in helping to restore function and health. Some techniques may be more effective for some people than others, and it is common for people to visit more than one chiropractor for their particular healthcare needs, depending on the chiropractor's specialty. Today, doctors of chiropractic are becoming more and more involved in workplace wellness programs and in whole-person preventive care. Readers interested in an in-depth overview of chiropractic history, theory, training, research, and clinical practice can read *Contemporary Chiropractic,* edited by Daniel Redwood, D.C., published by Churchill Livingstone. Another valuable reference is *The Chiropractic Profession* by David Chapman Smith, LLB (Hons). For additional information on chiropractic, contact the American Chiropractic Association at www.amerchiro.org or the International Chiropractic Association at www.chiropractic.org.

Dentistry (Holistic)

The American Holistic Dental Association was formed by a group of dentists who are interested in providing dental care that considers the condition of the gums, teeth, and mouth to be manifestations of the body's overall health, and they place great emphasis on care that is sensitive to the long-term effects of dental practices. It is important for you to be aware of the profound health effects of certain kinds of dental work, including bridge work, crowns, extractions, partials, and root canals.

One of the most important considerations in choosing a dentist is his or her attitude toward the use of amalgam fillings. These fillings contain large amounts of mercury, a highly toxic metal that is more poisonous than arsenic or lead. Although there is still debate in the American medical and dental community about the health effects of amalgam fillings, you deserve to know the truth about their potential for producing systemic mercury toxicity and significant harm to your health. Did you know that in numerous European countries, amalgam fillings are no longer being used? In fact, the government-sponsored health insurance program in Sweden encourages its citizens to have amalgam fillings removed and replaced with porcelain and other safer more acceptable materials.

Amalgam removal and replacement is a logical precaution for all health-conscious people. If you have one or more amalgam fillings in your teeth, consult with a holistically trained dentist about gradually replacing them, in order to maintain your general health and prevent possible neurological and immune-system disorders. For more information on whole-person dentistry, I encourage you to read *Whole Body Dentistry,* an outstanding book by holistic dentist Mark Breiner. Other excellent books on this controversial topic are *It's All in Your Head* by Hal Huggins, D.D.S., M.S.; *Silver Dental Fillings—The Toxic Time Bomb* by Sam Ziff; *Let the Tooth Be Known,* by Dawn Ewing, R.D.H., Ph.D., N.D.; and *The Oral Health Bible* by Michael Bonner, D.D.S. You may also wish to contact the Holistic Dental Association at www.holisticdental.org. This website can also help you find a holistically oriented and trained dentist in your area.

Homeopathy

The name homeopathy is derived from the Greek *homios* (similar) and *pathos* (suffering). This approach to health care was first identified by Samuel Hahnemann, M.D., whose early research demonstrated that in some cases, substances that produce specific symptoms in a healthy person could also cure the same set of symptoms in a sick person. Known as the law of similars, or like cures like, this idea was first expressed by the ancient Greek physician Hippocrates, the "Father of Medicine." In some ways, this theory was adapted for vaccinations, pioneered by Edward Jenner in his successful development of a smallpox vaccine. Homeopathy maintains that illness is a unique manifestation of a specific disease condition in a given patient. The symptoms a patient experiences are the body's best effort to maintain balance, equilibrium, and homeostasis. To the homeopathic physician, these symptoms provide a guide that directs the choice of the specific remedy for that specific disorder.

A wide range of plants, herbs, animal, and mineral sources make up the approximately 3,000 remedies used in homeopathic treatment. These remedies are diluted with distilled water and alcohol through a process called *potentization,* which actually makes the substances more potent—contrary to traditional scientific thought. In fact, most homeopathic remedies are diluted so much that none of the molecules from the original substance can be detected, even with the most sophisticated chemical analysis. Therefore, through the use of ultra small doses of medication, homeopathy can be considered a classic example of energy medicine, in the realm of vibrations, frequencies, and electromagnetic fields that have an effect on the body. Homeopathic remedies are among the safest substances in existence and are usually given in tablet form, as little pellets placed under the tongue, or as liquid drops also placed under the tongue.

Homeopathic remedies are carefully formulated to stimulate the body's innate vital force and, therefore, identifying the correct agent or combination of agents is an important process. First, the homeopathic practitioner obtains a detailed and lengthy patient history that considers medical as well as personal factors, such as emotional state, food choices, influences of the weather, and the person's belief system. Homeopathic doctors consider the whole person in their approach to care and attempt to prioritize the treatment starting with the area of the body most affected by illness, followed by less threatened areas of concern. Improvement occurs over a period of time, and there may even be a brief period when the patient's symptoms actually seem to get worse. To the homeopathic physician, however, this indicates that the healing process has begun and that rapid improvement will follow. As with most holistically oriented approaches, homeopathic practitioners emphasize a balanced emotional state, exercise, lifestyle, nutrition, and rest as part of an overall wellness program.

After decades of decline in use, homeopathy is currently enjoying a significant resurgence of popularity in the United States and most of the Western world. Over 500 million people receive homeopathic treatment every year throughout the world and it is generally considered a safe and intelligent choice for a wide variety of health concerns. Dana Ullman's *Discovering Homeopathy: Medicine for the 21st Century* is an informative, useful book on the subject.

Naturopathy

Before the era of sophisticated pharmacology and surgical techniques, ancient physicians had great respect for the healing power of nature. For example, the "Father of Medicine," Hippocrates, believed the body has the ability to heal itself when provided with pure air, water, and food, and given ample opportunity for exercise, the fundamental tools of natural healing. Thus naturopathy is histori- cally a part of virtually all systems of healing.

Naturopathic medicine became popular in European countries during the mid-nineteenth century. Benedict Lust was successfully treated with this natural approach to healing at the Father Sebastian Kneipp Health Spa, and in the 1890s, he introduced the broad-based teaching and practice of naturopathy to the United States. It has since become a separate, distinct system of healing, with its own schools and governmental regulations.

The naturopathic philosophy embraces the notion that illness results from chemical or metabolic stresses that are due to physical or emotional overloads on the body. Disease is considered the result of an overworked physical system that stresses and depresses the immune system. Naturopathic doctors place great emphasis on diet, frequently recommending specific foods and food combina- tions to aid the healing process, particularly organically grown fresh fruits and vegetables, nuts, seeds, whole grains, and pure water. To detoxify the body, naturopaths often recommend fasting, and strongly emphasize weight manage- ment and cleansing the body through methods such as colonic irrigation. Aro- matherapy, hydrotherapy, herbs, homeopathic remedies, massage, nutritional supplements, and a variety of stress reduction and relaxation techniques are also regularly prescribed by naturopaths.

Osteopathy

Traditional osteopathy was founded in the latter part of the nineteenth century by Andrew Taylor Still, M.D., who maintained that the body has the ability to heal itself if its structure is maintained and preserved. He believed that distur- bances in the body's framework could interfere with vital circulation to all the organs and systems of the body. Osteopathic treatment was originally applied by hand, using a combination of massage and manipulation of the joints. For approximately seventy-five years, its philosophy of care remained in keeping with that of its founder, who emphasized a non-drug, non-surgical approach to healing. However, today's osteopathic training and the scope of its practice have come to resemble conventional Western allopathic medicine, with an emphasis on pharmaceutical and surgical care in conjunction with traditional holistic considerations. Osteopathy is now widely recognized as a form of primary medical care, and doctors of osteopathy often practice many conventional medical sub-specialties.

Traditional osteopathy also has sub-specialties. Cranial osteopathy, founded by Dr. William Sutherland, and craniosacral therapy, founded by Dr. John Upledger, are manual care therapies that aim to maintain the flow of cerebrospinal fluid. Because they are very gentle, both treatments are often used on babies and children, particularly when there has been a history of birth trauma or childhood injury to the skull. These therapies are also used for adults with a wide variety of disorders that are difficult to diagnose and treat. Cranial osteopathy and craniosacral therapy are also practiced by some chiropractic physicians.

Psychiatry: A Critical Look

If you or someone you love is troubled by mental illness, you may be interested in learning about a more holistic approach to treating this family of disorders. For an objective, scientific assessment of the practice of psychiatry today read *Toxic Psychiatry* by Peter R. Breggin, M.D. Just consider the following statements taken from the book's jacket:

> "Prozac, Xanex, Halcion, Haldol, Lithium. These psychiatric drugs—and dozens of other short-term solutions—are being prescribed by doctors across the country as a quick antidote to depression, panic disorder, obsessive compulsive disorder, and other psychiatric problems. But, at what cost?

> "Psychiatrist Peter R. Breggin, M.D., breaks through the hype and false promises surrounding the new psychiatry and shows how dangerous and even potentially brain-damaging many of its drugs and treatments are. He asserts that psychiatric drugs are spreading an epidemic of long-term brain damage; mental illnesses like schizophrenia, depression, and anxiety disorder have never been proven to be genetic or even physical in origin, but are under the jurisdiction of medical doctors. Millions of children, housewives, older people, and others are labeled with medical diagnoses and treated with authoritarian interventions, rather than patiently listened to, understood and helped.

> "*Toxic Psychiatry* sounds a passionate, much-needed wake-up call for everyone who plays a part in America's ever increasing dependence

on harmful psychiatric drugs. Peter R. Breggin, M.D., is a leading critic of psychiatric drugs and the psychopharmaceutical complex. He is a graduate of Harvard College and Case Western Reserve Medical School and was formerly a teaching Fellow at Harvard Medical School and a full-time consultant with the National Institute of Mental Health. He is also the co-author, with Ginger Ross Breggin, of *Talking Back to Prozac;* and *The War Against Children,* published by St. Martin's Press."

Dr. Breggin also expresses his great concern about proper application of psychiatric drugs and warns his readers about the significant dangers of abruptly stopping their use, or using them without very careful medical supervision.

Psychotherapy

The term psychotherapy encompasses a broad range of treatments for mental, emotional, and related illnesses. Instead of relying on drug therapy, psychotherapists focus primarily on the patient's thoughts, emotions, and behaviors. Two of the best-known approaches, psychoanalysis and analytical psychotherapy, are patterned after the pioneering work of Austrian psychiatrist Sigmund Freud and Swiss psychiatrist Carl Jung. Cognitive behavior therapy, existential therapy, and humanistic psychotherapy are additional mental health tools used by doctors and therapists who are specially trained in the body/mind/spirit continuum of health. While most of these practitioners are not M.D. psychiatrists, they usually work with M.D.s and share many patient-care goals. Some psychologists and psychotherapists use a whole-person approach in managing mental health conditions, while others prefer to keep the various care disciplines separate and distinct. If you are interested in exploring psychotherapy as a treatment option, make sure that you are well-informed and take an assertive role in selecting your mental health clinician, just as you would in choosing any healthcare professional.

Orthomolecular Psychiatry by David R. Hawkins, M.D., Ph.D., with Nobel Laureate Linus Pauling, M.D., is an excellent book about the role of nutrition and environmental factors in mental health disturbances. It's a must-read for anyone who has a personal need, or has a family member with mental or emotional illness.

Voll Testing—Electro-Dermal Screening

A growing number of holistically oriented doctors and dentists are using an exciting energy-medicine technology known as electro-dermal screening, developed by Dr. Reinhold Voll, a German medical doctor, anatomy professor, and acupuncturist. Also referred to as electro-acupuncture by Voll (EAV), this is a highly sophisticated form of computerized energy analysis that is used to evaluate body functions and aids in the optimal application of botanical, homeopathic, and nutritional approaches. While electro-dermal screening has a wide range of applications, it is primarily used to detect allergies, environmental chemical exposure, heavy metal poisoning, and microbial infestation.

During electro-dermal screening, an imperceptible, low-voltage electrical charge is introduced into specific acupuncture points on the hands and feet. The goal of the procedure is to determine the precise amount of electrical current that is being conducted through each of the acupuncture meridian pathways of the body in order to discover energy imbalances. The level of the readings provides valuable information regarding the health and vitality of various organs and musculoskeletal regions of the body. Electro-dermal screening has proven extremely valuable to people struggling with a wide variety of acute and chronic health disorders, and is also very useful for general health maintenance.

Other Forms of Natural Healing

Additional forms of natural healing include art therapies, creative visualization, dance, humor, hypnotherapy, light and water therapies, music, play therapy, qigong, reiki, and Rolfing. Each method has its own unique application for healing and health maintenance. Qigong, reiki, and Rolfing are discussed in some detail below.

Qigong

Qigong is an ancient form of Chinese healing and meditation that combines special movements and controlled breathing. It is thought to improve the flow of the qi (ch'i) energy throughout the body. Visualization techniques to trace the meridian energy pathways and breath control are used to activate organ systems and improve the flow of circulation and facilitate detoxification. It is used in conjunction with other healing techniques and is especially helpful for stress-related conditions and those that involve the respiratory and circulatory systems.

Reiki

Reiki is an ancient form of hands on healing. Practitioners place their hands over specific parts of the body to direct energy to the patient's organs and systems in need. The goal of the therapy is to enhance the life force of the patient so that he or she can experience greater health and emotional harmony. It is used to physically energize the body and heal both chronic and acute disorders. Many practitioners also consider reiki a spiritual discipline that can transform both the patient and the healer.

Rolfing

Rolfing is a manual healing technique that emphasizes the importance of restoring the body's major components—the head, shoulders, thorax, pelvis, and legs—to an optimal vertical alignment. Rolfing is performed by practitioners who work on the muscles, fascia, and other connective tissues, using gentle, firm remolding forces that are applied by hand. The goal of the therapy is to gradually elongate the human frame and maintain its mass as close as possible over its vertical axis, thereby minimizing the amount of energy required to move the body through space. In addition to improved posture and appearance, overall organ and system function enhancement is also said to occur.

ASSOCIATIONS

In 1978, Norman Shealy, M.D., Ph.D., founded the American Holistic Medical Association, representing the principles and practices of holistic health care. Currently, the organization has approximately 1,000 members, and the number continues to grow. To learn more about the American Holistic Medical Association and to obtain the name and location of an AHMA member in your area, contact the organization at 1-505-292-7788 or visit their website at www.holisticmedicine.org. You may also wish to explore additional holistically oriented resources available through the American Holistic Nurses' Association. If you'd like to learn more, visit their informative website at www.ahna.org.

FIRST, DO NO HARM

Primum non nocera is a Latin phrase that all medical and healthcare students learn during their training. The literal translation is: First, do no harm. Another way of saying this is, "Remember that whatever you do to diagnose or treat your patients, do not harm them."

In the opening paragraph of this chapter, I suggested that your choice of healthcare practitioners—based upon their skill, experience, and attitude—could either save your life or threaten your life. It's important to recognize that there can be significant health risks involved in many diagnostic and treatment-related services. Indeed, some of these risks may even be life-threatening.

Consider the following article that appeared in the July 15, 1999, issue of the

Los Angeles Times headlined, "Kaiser CEO Injects Medical Safety Into Health care Debate." The article quoted a speech given by Dr. David Lawrence, Chief Executive of Kaiser Permanente, the nation's largest HMO, to the National Press Club:

"Medical accidents and mistakes kill 400,000 people a year, and rank only behind heart disease and cancer as the leading cause of death . . . . Mistakes alone kill more people each year than tobacco, alcohol, firearms, or automobiles. [Most patients] continue to believe in the myth of Marcus Welby, the unbridled benefits of technology, and the assumption that competence and safety are spread evenly and consistently throughout the healthcare system. If passengers were asked to fly with a commercial airline organized like most health care, they wouldn't get on the plane."

In addition, the Centers for Disease Control and Prevention (CDC) reports that hospital infections rates have risen 36 percent in the past twenty years. According to the CDC, of 35 million hospital admissions each year, 2.1 million patients will contract an infection from the hospital during their stay. Using data from a random sampling of 315 hospitals, the CDC estimates that 90,000 deaths from hospital infections occur every year, and it now ranks hospital germs as the fourth leading cause of death in the United States after heart disease, cancer, and strokes.

Whether you ultimately decide to try a natural approach to health care or choose to pursue a different path, you would be wise to pay careful attention to these statistics. By remaining vigilant, knowledgeable, and assertive as a health-care-services consumer, there is much you can do to avoid becoming an unfortunate casualty of the healthcare system. In considering any care providers, look for those who subscribe to a holistic point of view. The word physician means "healer," the word doctor means "teacher." Will your healthcare providers be willing to take the time to teach you and your loved ones the principles of healthy living? Will they genuinely listen to you and respect your insights, intelligence, and choices? Are their decisions regarding your care evaluated as much from their hearts as from their heads, hands, and computer readouts? Does your doctor have as much concern for your emotional and spiritual well-being as your physical health?

Openly Discuss the Care You Receive

If you are thinking of trying complementary, alternative therapies, it is important to discuss this with your primary care provider. Not doing so could actually have negative health consequences because of possible side effects and interactions between pharmaceutical drugs and herbal or botanical remedies recommended by natural healers. In addition, your primary care physician may order expensive diagnostic tests and procedures that have already been administered by other practitioners. Research by Harvard Medical School scientist David Eisenberg, M.D., and colleagues (1993 and 1997) found that of the millions of people who rely on unconventional therapies for their health problems, 72 percent are reluctant to discuss their use of alternative therapies with their primary care doctors. This is despite the fact that those who seek unconventional therapies generally had higher incomes and relatively more education. It seems that the majority of people who choose alternative treatments still believe their primary doctor will not understand or approve of this decision. Some also believe their doctors could refuse to care for them in the future after learning of their decision to receive care from an alternative healer.

In the past, physicians offering conventional care may have advised their patients to avoid alternative therapies and natural healing. Their reasoning was primarily based on perceptions that nonmedical doctors and other unconventional healthcare providers were inadequately trained to provide suitable diagnosis and care. Fortunately, these attitudes are rapidly changing, especially as training, licensing credentials, and other continuing educational standards continue to improve. In fact, independent research surveys show that more and more medical doctors (M.D.s) are regularly referring their patients to practitioners offering alternative healing. Additionally, hundreds of nonmedical doctors—including acupuncturists, chiropractors, herbal therapists, massage therapists, and naturopaths—are being invited to work in mainstream medical clinics. Since America is a consumer-driven society, this idea was advanced by the public's desire for healthcare providers to work together, and it is now in the process of becoming fully realized.

Alternative Forms of Care—Here to Stay

Dr. Eisenberg's studies show that, in 1990, Americans made an estimated 425 million visits to alternative therapists, such as acupuncturists and chiropractors—a number that well exceeds the approximately 388 million visits to all the primary care physicians in the United States put together. Of the sixteen most frequently used complementary or alternative therapies, Dr. Eisenberg found that relaxation techniques ranked number one, with 13 percent of the adult population seeking nonmedical approaches to relaxation and stress management. Ranked at number two was chiropractic care, with 10 percent of the adult population seeking this type of treatment. A 1997 follow-up to the 1990 study showed that instead of this being a passing fad, the number of people seeking complementary or alternative approaches to health care rose steadily in the seven years between the two studies, from approximately 34 percent in 1990 to about 42 percent by 1997.

Another such example is the increase in use of chiropractic care, which has doubled in the past twenty years throughout North America. The number of chiropractors has tripled since 1970, and will double again by 2010, and this trend is worldwide. Although chiropractic was founded in America, it is now practiced in over one hundred countries, and there are more chiropractic colleges outside the United States than within its borders. Studies have also shown that the great majority of people using alternative providers also consulted their primary physicians for the same or similar disorders. This being the case, I would recommend discussing complementary forms of care you are receiving with your primary care physician. You could be taking a big step toward assuring yourself safer, less expensive, and more comfortable care based on open communication and mutual respect. In addition, talking with your primary physician about your successful outcomes could enlighten him or her as to the value of such care; this could, in turn, help the doctor's other patients who might have health concerns similar to yours.

A worldwide shift in consciousness is now occurring in matters regarding health care and the human condition. This dramatic, historic happening can be compared with the peace and human rights movements around the time of the Vietnam War, and the environmental movement since. The new consciousness embraces a more balanced approach to true whole-person health care and demonstrates an appreciation for the innate, inner wisdom of the body to heal itself, as people are moving away from the crisis-oriented, damage-control, symptom-driven system of disease management known as contemporary health care. In this scenario, the best care may be the least care, and any care rendered is focused on the person rather than the disease. Ideally, doctors will essentially function as health "coaches" who will guide patients in determining what choices they should make to achieve and maintain excellent health.

These are exciting times. Congratulations on your decision to become an active participant in them.

THE PATIENT'S BILL OF RIGHTS

By being respectfully assertive with your doctors about all your healthcare needs, you will enjoy a healthier, longer, and more productive life. To this end, you should be aware of the American Hospital Association's "Patient's Bill of Rights," which states that you, as the patient, have the right to:

Be spoken to in words and phrases you understand

Be informed of your diagnosis

Full access to your medical records

Know the benefits and risks of all tests and treatments you are offered and any available alternatives

Know in advance the costs of all aspects of care

Share in all diagnostic and treatment decisions

Refuse any medical procedure

Obtain second and even third opinions from additional experts

Primary care physicians know and understand all the above and will usually encourage active participation in health and wellness goals. These rights apply to in-patient care in the hospital as well as outpatient services provided in a doctor's office or clinic. All healthcare providers must follow their established codes of ethics and scope of practice regulations. Your primary care physician cannot refuse to refer you to another specialist for a second opinion; likewise, any alternative healthcare provider who is treating you cannot refuse to refer you to appropriate conventional medical care when needed, especially in emergency situations. Should you ever feel your care provider has acted unprofessionally in these instances, you can write to your state's professional licensing agency.

HOW TO FIND A HOLISTICALLY ORIENTED MEDICAL DOCTOR

Most people who prefer alternative and complementary forms of healing are already under the care of a licensed professional who practices one or more approaches to nonpharmaceutical, noninvasive patient care. If you are already receiving some form of alternative or complementary health care, you may wish to ask your acupuncturist, chiropractor, nutritionist, massage therapist, or other natural practitioner for a referral to an open-minded, holistically oriented medical physician who will match your needs. If you are not currently using alternative healing methods, and you are trying to choose a primary care physician—family practice, internal medicine, or obstetrician/gynecologist—before you need her or his assistance with diagnosis or treatment. Be clear that the sole reason for your initial visit is to spend time learning about the practitioner's attitudes and beliefs toward your needs and concerns. If you feel awkward doing this, contact the American Holistic Medical Association or the American Holistic Nurses Association and ask for help in finding a holistically trained medical doctor in your area. Some doctors of chiropractic and osteopathy also function as primary care physicians or are members of an integrated team of care providers who offer holistically oriented forms of health care.

10. Don't Put Poisons into Your Body

his Golden Rule for the maintenance of your health has to do with avoiding the intake of poisons into your body. The healthy human body has an incredible ability to survive and even thrive, in spite of almost daily exposure to varying amounts of known toxic contaminants within the air we breathe, the water we drink, and the food we consume. This achievement is made possible by our bodies' innate ability to recognize the difference between things that are necessary and nourishing and in need of retaining, and things that are harmful and dangerous and in need of expelling. Perhaps the most astonishing thing is that it does this without our conscious awareness. The lungs have the ability to dispel the harmful carbon dioxide from our bodies and to retain the oxygen needed for life. The blood, lymph system, liver, kidneys, colon, and skin all work in harmony to discharge the toxic wastes from our bodies and do so with great efficiency. Obviously, however, there are *limits* on the amount and the potency of the toxins the body can effectively deal with and remain healthy. This chapter places emphasis on helping you understand the potential sources of subtle toxic exposure, such as heavy metals, fumes, and industrial and agricultural chemical hazards, and to encourage your avoidance of less subtle toxic agents, such as alcohol, tobacco, and drugs.

ALCOHOL

For most people, when used moderately and for the right purposes, small amounts of alcohol may be good for the body, mind, and spirit. In excess, however, alcohol is a depressant, and it can be toxic. Therefore, drink alcoholic beverages only in the way they are intended, for joyful, happy occasions, good times, and celebrations. Never drink alcohol when you're angry, depressed, lonely, or sad, and never use it in combination with drugs, including over-the-counter and prescription medications, and, most especially, antidepressant drugs.

Estimates from the Institute of Medicine of the National Academy of Sciences indicate that currently about 7 percent of Americans (nearly 14 million people) over the age of eighteen abuse alcohol or are addicted to alcohol. Alcohol contributes to 100,000 deaths each year, and 41 percent of all traffic fatalities are alcohol related. In addition, it is suggested that millions of people may be closet alcoholics—those who conceal their alcohol addiction from others. Among these individuals are homemakers, people living alone, retired people, self-employed people, and teenagers.

Sadly, statistics show that only one out of every eighteen known alcoholics eventually becomes sober and permanently avoids alcohol in the future, so prevention is clearly the key. How much alcohol is considered safe? Certain people seem to be highly sensitive and extremely vulnerable to alcohol abuse and addiction, and it is not presently known whether this predisposition has more to do with biological or psychological factors, or a combination of both. If you feel you might be one of the people at risk of developing alcoholism, particularly if you have a family history of the disease, you must totally avoid alcohol to prevent addiction. For most people of average size who are not as sensitive, any more than two ounces a day creates the potential for addiction. Each of the following contains one ounce of alcohol: one 12-ounce can of strong beer, one regular-size (wine) glass of wine, one highball or mixed drink containing one shot glass of whiskey, rum, vodka, gin, bourbon, or other liquor. Of course, this also depends on the alcohol content of the hard liquor. For example, if a whiskey is 100 proof, that means the product contains 50 percent pure alcohol; 80 proof means it is 40 percent alcohol, and so forth. Be aware of this, and be careful with your use of alcohol. It is known as the great deceiver, and its habit-forming effects are very subtle. Alcoholics can live in denial for years and years, often learning too late that their addiction has caused excessive, irreparable damage.

A special warning about alcohol during pregnancy: *No* amount is acceptable. Recent studies have shown that the brain of the growing fetus is especially vulnerable to the neurotoxic effects of alcohol, particularly during the last trimester. Fetal alcohol syndrome (FAS) has been linked to mental retardation, delayed growth, neurological damage, and behavioral disorders. Furthermore, if you are an alcoholic mother who has recently borne a child, and you are still drinking, do not breastfeed your baby, as your baby's brain and body tissues will absorb the alcohol through your breast milk and predispose your newborn to alcohol addiction with all its serious consequences.

Identifying Alcohol Abuse

The following can serve as a checklist for you or any family member who may be exhibiting these behavioral signs of alcoholism:

- An inability to stop at one or two drinks
- An inability to remember what occurred during a recent drinking bout
- An increased dependence on alcohol at social gatherings
- Becoming ill, vomiting, or passing out as a result of drinking alcohol
- Drinking alone
- Attempting to hide alcohol products at home or at work
- A gradual increase in the amount of alcohol consumed to effect a high
- Gulping down alcoholic beverages
- A regular neglect of personal appearance
- Family quarrels, tension, and arguments
- Tardiness in arriving home or at social engagements
- Changes in eating or sleeping habits
- Increased moodiness, irritability, or depression
- Hostile or aggressive behavior when drinking
- Attempts at concealing alcohol consumption with breath mints or mouthwash
- Repeated failed attempts to discontinue the use of alcohol
- Expressions of anger or denial regarding alcohol use and abuse
- A breakdown of personal or work relationships
- Shakiness that is relieved by alcohol consumption
- Using alibis and fabricating stories to cover drinking activity
- Absenteeism from work
- Drinking in the morning
- An inability to safely operate a motorized vehicle
- Overwhelming guilt for inappropriate behaviors while drinking

Possible Consequences of Alcohol Abuse

- Alcohol addiction
- Nutritional deficiency diseases

- Liver diseases such as cirrhosis or liver cancer
- Diseases affecting the pancreas, including cancer, diabetes, hypoglycemia, and pancreatitis
- Brain damage and neurological disorders
- Personality changes
- Gastric ulcers
- Heart disease, strokes, and blood clots
- Legal problems
- Employment problems
- Other compulsive behaviors, such as gambling, smoking, and drug abuse
- Social problems
- Vehicular accidents with potential fatalities and resultant felony charges, or prison terms
- Family and marital problems
- Broken homes and broken relationships
- Loneliness
- Depression
- Emotional, spiritual, and financial ruin

If alcohol abuse is impacting your life, listen to your inner spirit and make a decision to seek help. Join the millions who have chosen sobriety. Consult your phone book or search the Internet for a local chapter of Alcoholics Anonymous: their next lifesaving story could be your own. Because alcohol abuse is often associated with other forms of substance abuse, the consequences listed above could also be considered the same for all illicit or prescription-drug abuse and addiction. If you struggle with addiction to narcotics or other drugs, you can contact Narcotics Anonymous at www.na.org.

For friends and family members of people addicted to alcohol or drugs, involvement with Al-Anon can be a positive life-changing experience. You can learn more about the organization and find your local chapter at www.al-anon.alateen.org. The United Way's First Call for Help is also an important resource for people affected by all forms of substance abuse, or almost any personal or domestic problem. You can learn more by checking out their website at www.unitedway.org.

TOBACCO AND NICOTINE

Avoid tobacco in all of its forms. Nicotine and other substances contained in tobacco products are potent poisons that can have disastrous health consequences. The greatest risks of smoking and tobacco use are lung diseases, impaired circulation, heart attack, and impaired immunity. Additionally, smokers have twice the incidence of spine-related disorders as nonsmokers, and the incidence of degenerative disc disease in the neck joints is four times higher among tobacco users. And did you know that people who smoke have 50 percent more automobile accidents? It's true, and it's likely because they are distracted by the lighting up, flicking ashes, and snuffing out the butts in their ashtrays instead of keeping both hands available for safe driving. In fact, using tobacco products can increase your risk of developing almost every known disease, and results in premature wrinkling of the skin and sexual impotence. Recent studies indicate that teenagers who smoke are five times more likely to develop generalized anxiety, five times more likely to experience agoraphobia, and twelve times more likely to suffer from panic disorders.

As you can see, in addition to causing foul breath, body odor, and stained teeth and fingers, smoking is simply unhealthy, unglamorous, unintelligent, and unattractive. Use your common sense. Refuse to be a pawn of the money-mongering, death-peddling tobacco industry. Safe, effective, and affordable smoking cessation programs are widely available, and it's never too late to quit using tobacco, even if you have been a regular user for twenty years or more. Some smokers find it is easier to stop with a friend, co-worker, or spouse who smokes. The mutual support and challenge could make a real difference. Did you know that when you stop smoking, your risk of suffering a heart attack is cut in half within one year? And about five years after quitting, your risk is on par with someone who has never smoked.

Nicotine is a horribly addictive substance, but millions have managed to kick the habit, and 3,000,000 people quit each year. Just know in your heart you can do it, too—today, this week, this month. When you do decide to stop, remember that the worst cravings will be over in just a few days. The physical symptoms of withdrawal may last for a couple of weeks, but after that it's all psychological. Don't delay. If you genuinely care about yourself, just do it.

The Dangers of Secondhand Smoke

Even if you don't smoke, cigarette smoking can be a danger to your health. Secondhand smoke can increase your risk of developing many of the same diseases that affect smokers. Consider the following statistics provided by The American Cancer Society, The American Heart Association, The Centers for Disease Control, The Irish Cancer Society, *The Journal of the American Medical Association (JAMA),* The National Research Council, and The World Health Organization:

- It is estimated that only 15 percent of cigarette smoke is inhaled by the smoker. The remaining 85 percent, which contains forty-three cancer-causing agents and 200 poisons, lingers in the air for everyone else to breathe as secondhand smoke.

- A non-smoking woman whose husband smokes on a regular basis has a 91 percent greater risk of developing heart disease. This same woman will have twice the risk of dying from lung cancer.

- Children whose parents both smoke can inhale the equivalent of 102 packs of cigarettes by age five.

- Infants whose parents both smoke at home are four times more likely to die from sudden infant death syndrome (SIDS).

- Children whose parents smoke have a greater incidence of asthma, bronchitis, ear infections, and pneumonia. They also miss more school and are hospitalized more often.

After considering the above, if you care about the people close to you and you still choose to continue smoking, do the right thing and smoke outdoors. If you have friends or loved ones who smoke, share what you've learned with them and urge them to smoke outdoors, or leave the room if they smoke indoors.

ILLEGAL, PRESCRIPTION, AND OVER-THE-COUNTER DRUGS

All illicit drugs, including marijuana, are toxic and cause significant, sometimes irreversible harm to the body, mind, and spirit. Thus, commonsense dictates that you should not experiment with these substances under any circumstances. Even prescription drugs should be used with great care and awareness. In 1995, the Food and Drug Administration (FDA) reported that 141,000 deaths that year were caused by adverse reactions to prescription drugs. J. Lyle Bootman, Dean of the University of Arizona College of Pharmacy, told The American Medical Association's 14th Annual Science Reporters Conference in October of 1995 that, "We spend approximately $75 billion for [pharmaceutical] drugs annually and another $76 billion for problems caused by drugs and the treatments."

Another fifteen to twenty thousand deaths are now attributed to over-the-counter (OTC) products, primarily the non-steroidal anti-inflammatory drugs (NSAIDs) such as aspirin and non-aspirin compounds used for headaches, mild fevers, and joint and muscle pain. The primary cause of death from NSAIDs is uncontrolled bleeding of the stomach and gastrointestinal tract, a common side effect of these heavily advertised products. Another known side effect of these OTC products is kidney damage, which is irreversible in most cases. Did you know that if you are between the ages of twenty-five and sixty-four, taking just two aspirin tablets a day increases your chances of kidney disease by 900 percent? A recent article in the medical journal *Neurology* reported that people who used Lipitor, Pravachol, Zocor, or other prescribed cholesterol-lowering statin drugs for two or more years were twenty-six times more likely to develop a condition known as idiopathic polyneuropathy, a painful disorder that causes inflammation of all the nerves of the body.

The best thing you can do for yourself to avoid any health risks from prescription and OTC medications is to become educated about all of the medications you take. If you take any prescription drugs regularly ask your prescribing doctor or your pharmacist about any potentially dangerous interactions with other medications or herbal remedies. Also ask about any side effects that may occur if you drink grapefruit juice because it can cause the concentration of many drugs to reach dangerously toxic levels, for reasons that are not yet fully understood.

Additionally, request a full explanatory printout of any medication you are taking when you pick up the prescription and read this information carefully. If you do not understand some of the technical words, look them up or ask your pharmacist what they mean. If they're not too busy, most professionals are happy to take time to dispense advice. Do this for your health as well as for your family's health and protection.

ARE VACCINATIONS SAFE?

The American Academy of Pediatrics currently recommends twenty-one vaccinations for children by the time they are in first grade. Most American pediatricians and government-sponsored health agencies wholeheartedly support this practice. Likewise, adults—particularly those serving in the armed forces—are subjected to a battery of immunizations intended to prevent a variety of illnesses.

For the most part, vaccinations have a positive track record. They drastically lower the incidence of contagious diseases, saving up to 30,000 lives each year, and they are considered statistically safe. However, some organizations continue to raise serious questions regarding the safety and efficacy of these mandatory public health practices. They point out vaccination-related links to a variety of health conditions, including immune system disturbances, learning disorders, medication-resistant seizures, mental retardation, paralysis, and death. Could all these concerns of trained, intelligent individuals be based solely on hysteria? How much of the resistance to mandatory vaccination programs should be considered exaggerated and non-scientific?

While some concerns about the risks of vaccinations still exist, particularly with smallpox and anthrax vaccines, great strides have been made in the manufacture, storage, distribution, safety, and efficacy of most vaccines, particularly in recent years. The Centers for Disease Control National Immunization Program website, www.cdc.gov/nip, lists the U.S. government's vaccination recommendations for infants, children, and adults. To learn more about case studies and critical concerns expressed by the National Vaccine Information Center, check out the NVIC website at www.nvic.org.

If you would like further information on alternative considerations in childcare and effective preventive measures, there are a number of excellent books available, including *How to Raise a Healthy Child in Spite of Your Doctor* and *Immunizations: The Terrible Risks Your Children Face That Your Doctor Won't Reveal,* both by well-known pediatrician Robert Mendelsohn, M.D. While significant improvements in public inoculation programs have been made since these two books were first published, Dr. Mendelsohn's voice and commentary on immunization in particular and childcare in general are still enlightening parents. I also recommend *Vaccinations* by Aviva Jill Romm, *What Every Parent Should Know About Childhood Immunization* by Jamie Murphy and Carol White, and *What Your Doctor May Not Tell You About Children's Vaccinations* by Stephanie Cave and Deborah Mitchell. Each of these books provides well-researched, candid commentary on this highly sensitive and controversial topic.

HEAVY METAL TOXICITY

Heavy metal toxicity may be at the root of more chronic diseases than we know, because many people are not even aware of its prevalence. Conditions such as anemia, arthritis, attention deficit disorder (ADD), brain damage, depression, digestive problems, fatigue (including chronic fatigue syndrome), glandular imbalances, and osteoporosis are regularly seen in people with heavy metal poisoning. Most of the time it's difficult to diagnose heavy metal toxicity because the body disposes of toxins through the excretory system, including the kidneys, bowels, skin, and so forth, and the residuals remain in the blood for only a short time after exposure. If the exposure is continuous, however, and the body is unable to fully eliminate heavy metal toxins, they are stored in the bones, brain, fatty tissues, glands, and nerves. The most reliable means of detecting heavy metal toxicity is with a chelating agent, a special preparation that binds to the heavy metal so that it can be eliminated through the urine. After the chelating agent is ingested, the urine can be tested for the presence of heavy metals. Another method testing for heavy metal toxicity is electro-dermal screening (EDS), which is described on page 60.

The treatment for heavy metal poisoning usually involves supplementing chelation therapy with herbs, homeopathy, and nutrients such as vitamin C. Drinking lots of fresh, pure water helps to detoxify the body, as do exercise, saunas, and steam baths, all of which induce sweating that enables the body to release toxins through the skin. Fiber-rich vegetables, especially broccoli, cabbage, and cauliflower, can aid the detoxification process, too, as can garlic and onions.

Some of the heavy metals that most commonly cause toxicity are discussed below.

Aluminum

Exposure to any more than trace amounts of aluminum can be toxic. Diseases believed to be related to aluminum toxicity include Alzheimer's disease, breast cancer, and lymphoma. Aluminum is found in many antacids used for indigestion, and in several underarm antiperspirants. Because toxins from aluminum cookware and aluminum foil can leach into foods, you should avoid using these products entirely, and instead choose glass, stainless steel, or high-grade stoneware for cooking and storing your food.

Mercury

Mercury is among the most toxic substances found in nature. We first discussed mercury toxicity in Chapter 9 as it relates to amalgam dental fillings. In the past decade or so, we have also become aware that many of our lakes and streams have been contaminated by mercury and a variety of other toxic chemical and industrial wastes. Warnings about eating fish caught from contaminated waterways continue to be issued by state departments of health and various other government agencies, and they are not to be taken lightly.

It's also possible to experience mercury poisoning if you accidentally break an oral thermometer containing the element. Should this happen, keep your distance from the spilled mercury so that you do not breathe the vapors or allow the substance to touch your skin. Contact the Poison Control Center at 1-800-222-1222 to find out the appropriate way to dispose of the spilled mercury. Do not sweep it up and throw it into the trash, because this is not only hazardous to your health, but it can also be hazardous to the environment, since mercury can find its way into the soil, the groundwater, and eventually the food chain.

A lesser-known source of mercury toxicity, particularly in infants and children, is the mercury-based vaccine preservative Thimerosal, manufactured by Eli Lilly and Company. Since this product has been in widespread use since the 1930s, it's possible that people of all ages may have residual amounts of mercury in their systems. Today, a growing number of cases are in litigation involving infants who have serious neurological illness and injuries from the Thimerosol contained in their pediatric vaccines.

Lead

It's estimated that the average person living today has 500 times more lead in his or her body than someone who lived in the Middle Ages. The two most common sources of lead poisoning are lead-based paints and leaded plumbing materials—both of which are still found in some older houses, office buildings, and factories. In the case of plumbing, drinking and cooking water can become contaminated and very hazardous to anyone who is exposed to it. Other sources of lead poisoning are certain types of handmade pottery used for cooking and food storage. Where still used, leaded gasoline also poses a danger. And, in fact, lawns and playgrounds adjacent to busy streets and highways may still be contaminated with residual poisons from lead-rich exhaust spewed by millions of vehicles that passed nearby in the years when leaded gasoline was the standard in much of the world.

Children are most at risk for lead poisoning. Symptoms may include delayed intelligence, behavioral disorders, reading difficulties, impaired hand-eye coordination, delayed growth, and nervous system disorders. For children and adults, exposure to lead accumulation in the body can result in damage to the kidneys, heart, liver, and nervous system. Over time, the gums turn blue and the patient may suffer notable muscle weakness. Eventually, lead poisoning can result in blindness, paralysis, loss of memory, personality disorders, and reproductive dysfunction.

If your home was built before 1930, lead pipes may have been used in the plumbing. In homes built prior to the mid-1980s, copper pipes were joined with lead-based solder, which still resulted in lead leaching into drinking, bathing, and cooking water supplies. If either of these conditions exists in your home, you may need to replace the plumbing to permanently overcome the hazard. Banned since 1986, the use of copper pipes soldered with lead has been replaced by the use of plastic and other synthetic materials that do not require lead sealants.

Older homes may also have woodwork that was covered with lead-based paints. This can be particularly dangerous for babies and toddlers who may suck or chew on painted surfaces, such as windowsills, or eat chips that have broken free. Old painted wooden baby cribs and playpens may pose a similar hazard.

Cadmium

Cadmium toxicity can result from prolonged exposure to cigarette smoke, the manufacture of plastics, and working around nickel-cadmium batteries and some red oil paints. It is also sometimes found in fertilizers, fungicides, pesticides, coffee, tea, and soft drinks.

Symptoms of cadmium poisoning include loss of the sense of smell, anemia, hair loss, dry skin, loss of appetite, and high blood pressure. It has also been associated with liver and kidney disease, cancer, and a diminished immune system.

Ask your healthcare provider about investigating the possibility of cadmium toxicity if you think you have been exposed.

Fluoride

Fluoride is more toxic than lead, and even in extremely small amounts, it can damage the brains and nervous system of a developing child. Some evidence also connects fluoride toxicity with conditions such as arthritis, cancer, excessive bone fractures, and genetic defects. In light of these factors, you may be surprised to know that fluoride is still added to commercial water supplies in most U.S. cities, although there has always been a great deal of controversy surrounding this practice. For example, the Food and Drug Administration (FDA) has taken the position that fluoride added to the water supply is not a mineral nutrient but rather a prescription drug. Because all prescription drugs have potential side effects, the FDA has never approved fluoride for use in the public water supply. Likewise, the Environmental Protection Agency (EPA) has concluded, after studying all the evidence for and against fluoridation, that the public water supply should not be used "as a vehicle for disseminating this toxic and pro-phylactically [intended for prevention] useless substance."

Most developed countries have either stopped adding fluoride to public water sources or never engaged in this practice at all because it's impossible to control the amount individuals may consume. In the United States, the wide-spread use of fluoride in public water supplies, dental products, foods, and beverages made with ingredients grown with fluoridated water or bottled with it poses a real danger of overexposure and toxicity. While the American Dental Association (ADA) continues to advocate the use of fluoride in public water supplies, many respected doctors, health scientists, and some dentists are against adding fluoride to city water supplies. You can learn more about the highly contested issue of fluoridation at the Fluoride Action Network's website at www.fluoridealert.org.

Arsenic

While not technically a heavy metal, arsenic is an extremely poisonous semi-metallic element that exists naturally in our environment and should be considered in the evaluation of health disorders—especially blood diseases, heart disease, high blood pressure, lung cancer, and various types of nerve damage. Arsenic compounds are used in the manufacture of pharmaceuticals, glass, fungicides, herbicides, and pesticides, and in tanning products, taxidermy preservatives, and textile printing. Carpenters, woodworkers and people working in the lumber industry should also be aware that wood preservatives used in the production of chemically treated, life-extending lumber may contain potentially dangerous levels of arsenic.

ASPARTAME

Aspartame is a very popular chemical used as an artificial sweetener and substitute for table sugar—and it's considered toxic and harmful to human health. In 1995, the U.S. Food and Drug Administration documented over ninety symptoms and adverse physical, mental, and emotional reactions attributed to the use of aspartame. I strongly recommend entirely avoiding products that contain this chemical. This may not be easy, however, as almost 5,000 food and medicinal products currently contain aspartame, including diet drinks and diet foods, so you should carefully review food labels to see if it's listed as an ingredient.

For an understanding of the neurotoxic nature of aspartame, as well as the negative health effects of the flavor-enhancing chemical monosodium glutamate (MSG), I recommend reading *Excitotoxins: The Taste That Kills* by neurosurgeon Russell Blaylock, M.D.

HOUSEHOLD CLEANERS, SOLVENTS, AND PERSONAL CARE PRODUCTS

It's important to be cautious about your use of household products such as herbicides, insect sprays, lawn and garden products, paints, rodent controls, solvents, and more. You may be surprised to learn that many of these products actually contain poisons and carcinogens (cancer-causing agents). For example, the label on many brands of toothpaste state, "Keep out of the reach of children under 6 years of age. If you accidentally swallow more than used for brushing, seek professional help or contact a poison control center immediately." Check the label of your own brand of toothpaste and you may find a similar warning.

In the interest of your health, you may wish to patronize health food stores and the natural foods and products section of your grocery store. And don't be bashful about asking retail stores for nontoxic products. I also recommend looking into Neways International, a company that specializes in excellent nontoxic personal care and homecare products. You can find them on the Internet at www.neways.com.

ADDITIONAL TOXIC SUBSTANCES

Although there have been 70,000 to 80,000 new chemicals introduced into our environment in the past hundred years, only about 1,500 of these substances have ever been tested for safety, and almost none of them have been tested in combination with other agents. In addition, only about 30 percent of the 17,000 chemicals commonly found in household cleaning and personal care products have been tested for health and safety. Manufacturers are not required to label the exact ingredients of these products, so the consumer is left totally unaware of any toxic or carcinogenic effects.

Understanding these facts helps us realize that many more dangerous heavy metals and toxic chemicals than we realize regularly find their way into products we use everyday, as well as into our air, food, and water sources. Some of the hundreds of toxic substances are asbestos; benzene; beryllium; DDT; formaldehyde; methyl chloride; paraquat, known as agent orange; and radon, a radioactive toxic gas resulting from the breakdown of radium. If you have questions or concerns about environmental toxins that may be affecting your health, contact The Agency for Toxic Substances and Disease Registry, listed in the Resources section in the back of this book.

11. Heart Disease and Stroke

Cardiovascular disease, affecting the heart and blood vessels, is the number-one killer in America today. Heart attacks and strokes kill almost 1,000,000 people every year, and more people die from coronary heart disease and strokes than all other causes of death combined. Currently, 63 million Americans (about 25 percent) have some form of cardiovascular disease.

By far, the major cause of heart attack and stroke is inflammation and hardening of the arteries, which results in a buildup of hard, fatty plaque deposits on the inner lining of blood vessels that supply nutrients and oxygen to the heart and the brain. There are many different factors that contribute to the blockage, breakdown, hardening, and inflammation of these critically important blood vessels.

The Golden Rules outlined in this chapter will provide important information to help you avoid becoming a casualty of the most fatal health disorder known to humans.

UNCONTROLLABLE FACTORS IN CARDIOVASCULAR DISEASE

Although age, gender, race, and family history are factors beyond our control, they all contribute to the potential for heart attacks and strokes. Of these, perhaps the single greatest predictor of developing heart and blood-vessel diseases is a family history of these conditions. Therefore, if your parents, grandparents, uncles, and aunts have a high incidence of cardiovascular illnesses, chances are high that you're also at risk. Obviously, you can't choose your ancestors, but there are preventive measures you can take to protect your health.

CONTROLLABLE FACTORS— LIFESTYLE CHOICES DO MATTER

The controllable factors in heart attack and stroke are numerous and include smoking and tobacco use, alcohol consumption, chronic dehydration, poor diet, diabetes, high blood pressure, high cholesterol levels, lack of exercise, and stress. Making positive lifestyle choices, as outlined here and throughout this book, can greatly increase your chances of living a longer, healthier life.

Food Choices and Cooking Habits

Beginning with food, a major step toward helping to prevent heart attacks, strokes, hardening of the arteries, and a wide variety of other blood-vessel diseases is to cut out animal fats and foods fried in animal fats from your diet. On the other hand, lean red meats, especially if not overcooked, can actually be beneficial in the prevention of cardiovascular diseases, as they contain many essential nutrients that are not as widely available in other foods. It's better to bake, broil, or steam your foods and always avoid overcooking. Also, refer back to Chapter 4 for a list of foods that will help keep your body chemistry alkaline.

Choosing Your Fats and Oils

One very important measure to take in preventing coronary artery heart disease, is to avoid using saturated fat products, such as lard and excessive amounts of butter. You should also avoid semi-solid vegetable oil products, including margarine and Crisco. In fact, Crisco is made from palm oil, one of the oils highest in saturated fat. When you use oils for baking, cooking, or salad dressings, extra virgin olive oil is best. Canola oil, or rapeseed oil, is also generally a healthy choice, unless it's from genetically engineered sources, so remember to choose a certified organic brand. Although liquid vegetable oils such as corn, safflower, and soybean oils contain less saturated fat than solid vegetable oil products and animal fats, including them in your diet can contribute significantly to your total fat intake. The average adult needs only about 14 grams of fat—less than a tablespoon—each day to take in healthy amounts of essential fatty acids, but the average American consumes almost *eight times* the recommended maximum. Including saturated fats or an excessive amount of monounsaturated and polyunsaturated fats in your diet will gradually elevate your cholesterol and significantly increase your risk of developing hardening of the arteries.

Avoid Hydrogenated Fats and Oils

Avoid any product that contains hydrogenated or partially hydrogenated oils. Hydrogenation is a stage of food processing that's done exclusively to increase a product's shelf life by making the oils more saturated. What the label will not tell you however, is that this process will also increase your risk for developing coronary artery disease.

Healthful Sources of Essential Fats and Oils

The body requires about 14 grams of essential fatty acids (EFAs) daily not only to maintain general health, but also for optimal cardiovascular health. Good sources of EFAs include vegetable oils, such as olive, flax, sesame, and primrose oils. (Remember to select organically produced oils whenever you can find them!) Other excellent sources of essential fatty acids are coldwater ocean fish, including cod, halibut, herring, mackerel, salmon, sardines, and tuna. However, because some ocean waters have become contaminated with arsenic or mercury, which can build up in the meat of fish, plant sources of EFAs are the preferred choice. Vegetable oils such as those listed above can be added to salad dressings or blended into fruit smoothies. I recommend Udo's Choice Perfected Oil Blend of unrefined oils, which contains the balanced ratio of omega 3, omega 6 and omega 9 oils important for optimal health. Some oils must be refrigerated to prevent rancidity, so read labels carefully when you're choosing these products. It's important to note, however, that all essential oil products have a limited window of time during which they can be safely consumed.

Helpful Supplementation

Including soy lecithin, garlic, vitamins E, C, and plenty of B vitamins—particularly vitamin B_6 and folic acid—in your daily diet can also be an excellent means of reducing your risk for hardening of the arteries, heart attack, high blood pressure, and stroke.

Recent studies have shown that perhaps one of the highest risk factors for heart attack is the level of an amino acid called homocysteine in the bloodstream. Fortunately, supplementing with as little as 500 micrograms (mcg) of folic acid and 50 mg of vitamin B_6 daily can effectively reduce levels of homocysteine. To learn more about the link between homocysteine and heart disease and the importance of B vitamins in heart health, I recommend reading *The Homocysteine Revolution* by Kilmer McCully, M.D.

C-Reactive Protein

Most people are aware that high cholesterol is a significant factor in hardening of the coronary arteries. But it's important to know that half of all the 1.1 million heart attacks reported annually occur in people whose blood fats are at normal levels. Recent studies have shown that a painless inflammation of the blood-vessel walls may increase the risk of heart attack and other diseases that affect the blood vessels, such as strokes. This inflammation weakens the walls of blood vessels, allowing built-up plaque and fatty deposits to break loose and cause a heart attack.

Fortunately, appropriate testing can detect this inflammatory condition. Abnormal levels of C-reactive protein in your blood signify a generalized acidic, inflammatory condition in the body that can lead to heart attack and stroke. If your doctor finds that you have high C-reactive protein levels, you would be wise to keep your body chemistry alkaline through dietary choices, as recommended in Chapter 4; reduce stress in your life; and follow the lifestyle modifications recommended throughout this book.

Too Much or Not Enough?

High blood pressure, high cholesterol, hardening of the arteries, heart attack, and stroke are frequently caused or aggravated by:

Too much salt (sodium chloride), not enough potassium

Too much phosphorous, not enough calcium and magnesium

Too much sugar and refined starches, not enough fruits, vegetables, and nuts

Too much sedentary activity, too little exercise

Too much coffee, tea, soda, and alcohol, not enough pure water

Too much animal fat in the diet, not enough essential vegetable and fish oils

Too much nicotine and carbon monoxide, not enough fresh air

Too much stress, hustle-bustle, and hassle, not enough deep relaxation

Too much anger, bitterness, and resentment, not enough forgiveness and tolerance

Too much loneliness, isolation, not enough affection and appreciation

Too much selfishness, not enough sharing and giving

Too much emphasis on pleasure, not enough emphasis on happiness

Too much anxiety, fear, and worry, not enough trust and faith

STEPS TO TAKE IF YOU ARE SUFFERING A HEART ATTACK

What should you do if you are alone and you feel you may be experiencing signs of a heart attack? Symptoms of a heart attack include sudden shortness of breath with severe chest pain that radiates into your left shoulder and arm, tightness and pain between your shoulder blades, or a pain in your jaw. Without immediate medical assistance, most people have a very short time before they could begin to lose consciousness and, too often, die. If you find yourself in this situation and you have access to a telephone, immediately dial 911 and then try intentionally coughing deeply and vigorously. For some, this simple action is lifesaving. Before each cough, take a deep breath, and continue coughing about every two seconds until emergency help arrives or you arrive at the emergency room. Deep breaths send oxygen to the lungs, and the sharp movements of the rib cage from coughing squeeze the heart muscle to help keep blood circulating. Even if the pain subsides and your heartbeat returns to what seems normal, you still must follow up with a medical professional to determine what treatment and lifestyle changes you require to maintain or improve your health.

Important note: If a person who is driving experiences symptoms of an impending heart attack, he or she should immediately pull the vehicle over to the side of the road, as a loss of consciousness while driving could pose a serious risk to the driver and to others.

STROKES: AGE IS NOT NECESSARILY THE MOST IMPORTANT FACTOR

Each year, approximately 600,000 Americans suffer strokes—either their first stroke or a recurrent episode. While the risk of stroke doubles each decade after age thirty-five, it may surprise you to learn that each year an estimated 25,000 relatively young American men and women in their thirties and forties suffer strokes. For people in this age group, strokes often result from a blockage of oxygenated blood to the brain, and are secondary to a clot or plaque buildup in the arteries that feed nutrients and oxygen to the brain. A smaller number of strokes result from a ruptured blood vessel within the brain. While many of the risk factors for heart attack are the same for stroke, men are much more vulnerable to strokes than women because more men smoke and are less likely to schedule checkups for high blood pressure, high cholesterol, or diabetes.

Warning Signs of Stroke

- Sudden, severe headache with no apparent cause.

- Sudden, unexplained numbness, weakness, or paralysis of the face, arms or legs, especially if on one side of the body.

- Abrupt loss of speech, slurring, or difficulty talking or understanding the speech of others.

- An immediate loss of vision in one or both eyes.

- Unexplained dizziness or unsteadiness that may cause you to fall, especially with any of the symptoms listed previously.

If you or someone in your presence experiences one or more of these warning signals, call 911 immediately. Prompt emergency treatment has saved many lives and can greatly reduce the long-term effects of stroke, including brain damage. If the stroke is caused by a blood clot, a new drug called t-PA has been proven effective in reducing brain damage if it's administered within three hours of the stroke. For further information on strokes and their prevention, visit the National Stroke Association's website at www.stroke.org.

SUMMARY

Information about heart disease and stroke prevention and treatment could easily take up several chapters in this book, but I have chosen to keep this chapter reasonably short, and simply to provide basic, essential information. Following the Golden Rules provided in this book will help keep you healthy and protect you against heart attack or stroke. However, if you have already been diagnosed with a heart or vascular disease or you have a strong hereditary predisposition to any of the conditions highlighted in this chapter, the basic information presented here may not be adequate for your needs. Should you find that you need more help in improving your cardiovascular health, I strongly recommend that you read *Dr. Dean Ornish's Program for Reversing Heart Disease: The Only System Scientifically Proved to Reverse Heart Disease without Drugs or Surgery.* It's an absolutely wonderful book that is enlightening as well as entertaining— and it just may save your life. The following are excerpts from the book jacket of Dr. Ornish's:

> This is a book about healing your heart. In this breakthrough book, Dr. Dean Ornish presents the first scientific proof that it is possible to actually reverse heart disease without drugs or surgery.
>
> Dr. Ornish's internationally acclaimed scientific study, funded in part by the National Institutes of Health and based on thirteen years of research, has yielded astonishing conclusions: Heart disease can be halted or even reversed—without bypass surgery, angioplasty or cholesterol lowering drugs—simply by changing our lifestyle.

Participants in Dr. Ornish's study, all of whom had severe coronary heart disease, followed his extraordinary Opening Your Heart program with amazing results: their chest pain diminished or disappeared; they often were able to reduce or discontinue medications; they felt more energetic, happy, and calm; they lost weight while eating much more food; and in most cases the average blockages in their coronary arteries began to reverse. In fact, the more severely blocked arteries showed the most reversal.

In contrast, the coronary blockages of most of the patients who followed their (regular) doctors' recommendations became worse instead of better.

Even more prevalent than physical heart disease are the psychological and spiritual diseases of the heart; loneliness and isolation from each other, and from the higher parts of ourselves. We can learn how to open our hearts on emotional and spiritual levels as well as anatomical ones. Ultimately, the Opening Your Heart program is about learning how to feel freer and happier—a different type of "open-heart" procedure, one based on love, knowledge, and compassion rather than just drugs and surgery.

And Larry Dossey, M.D., author of *Space, Time, and Medicine* and *Recovering the Soul* said this regarding Dr. Ornish's book:

This is an epochal book. It sets a new standard in our understanding of heart disease, and it is the template against which all other books on any disease whatsoever should be judged. For the purity of the science on which it rests, and for the majesty of its spiritual wisdom, this book has no equal in the literature of medicine and health.

Hopefully these words will stimulate your curiosity about this extraordinary, holistically oriented book. Thank you, Dr. Ornish, for providing the world with this lifesaving information and inspiration.

12. Blood Sugar Disorders

efined sugars and processed starches included in excess in your diet place stress on your body that can result in blood sugar disorders such as diabetes and hypoglycemia. Drinking alcohol and caffeinated beverages and consuming high-fat foods only increases the risk of developing these conditions. If your diet is less than healthy and particularly if you have a family history of hypoglycemia and diabetes, you need to be especially vigilant about managing your diet and watching for signs that you may be developing problems with blood sugar.

DIABETES MELLITUS

There are two primary types of diabetes mellitus, each having their own characteristics, as discussed below.

Type I Diabetes Mellitus

Type I diabetes is also known as insulin-dependent diabetes or juvenile diabetes. The reason for this distinction is that it usually strikes during childhood or young adulthood, and most often requires insulin therapy immediately upon diagnosis and thereafter throughout one's life. The predominant symptoms of type I diabetes are:

- Excessive hunger
- Excessive thirst
- Fatigue
- Frequent urination

- Irritability
- Nausea and vomiting
- Weakness

Type II Diabetes Mellitus

Type II diabetes is also known as adult-onset (or maturity-onset) diabetes. It is commonly found in people with a family history of the disorder. Dietary measures and exercise are often sufficient in controlling this type of diabetes; however, if neglected or poorly managed, it can result in devastating outcomes that include blindness and severe loss of circulation to the limbs, sometimes requiring amputation. The classic signs and symptoms of type II diabetes are:

- Blurred vision

- Dry, itchy skin

- Excessive thirst

- Excessive urination

- History of obesity with recent weight loss

- Increased appetite

- Increased food consumption

- Loss of strength and endurance

- Mood swings

- Slow healing of cuts and wounds

- Tingling or numbness of the hands and feet

The cost of care for diabetes in America exceeds 100 billion dollars each year. It is a very serious disorder that, if left uncontrolled, can have grave consequences, including blindness, neurological disorders, kidney disease, and loss of circulation to the lower extremities that can lead to gangrene requiring amputation. Undiagnosed and untreated, diabetes can eventually result in coma and even death. Did you know that people with diabetes have four times more heart attacks than people who don't have the disorder, and are much more likely to die as the result of a heart attack? Do whatever you can to prevent this condition, and if you already have diabetes, do your very best to prevent or minimize the complications.

The majority of those with advanced diabetes require insulin replacement therapy. (There are, however, millions of people with type II diabetes who can completely control their blood-sugar levels without insulin replacement therapy, simply by modifying their diet, exercising, and making lifestyle changes.) Less severe diabetes or other blood sugar disorders can usually be stabilized effectively with lifestyle and dietary changes. Many people with either high or low blood sugar find great therapeutic value in calcium, chromium, magnesium, and zinc supplements, and including garlic, Jerusalem artichokes, and onions in the diet. Some chiropractors have reported that their patients require less insulin following structural manual care aimed at balancing the nervous, endocrine, and digestive systems of the body. If you haven't explored these simple, inexpensive, all-natural approaches, you may be amazed to learn that they have the potential to be so effective. As with any treatment program, however, it's very important that you continue to carefully monitor your blood glucose levels and see your doctor regularly because the results can be dramatic, and you may need to adjust your insulin intake.

Children Are at Great Risk

Probably the population at greatest risk for type II diabetes in today's society are children whose diets have consisted primarily of refined starches, sugars, and saturated fats. Childhood obesity is now reaching alarming rates in the United States, as more and more children consume Mountain Dew and Twinkies for breakfast, macaroni and cheese for lunch, and Coke and pizza for dinner. Usually the first indication of such nutritional abuse is excessive weight, including obesity; behavioral disorders; mood swings, anxiety, and depression; and fatigue. Many of these high-fat, high-sugar foods and beverages are also laced with significant amounts of artificial colorings, flavorings, and preservatives that can greatly disturb the body's health and harmony. Today it is more common to find children as young as ten years of age being diagnosed with type II diabetes, formerly known as adult onset diabetes because it generally affected people in their forties and beyond. Obviously, parents of growing children should take note of this important information so they can keep their kids healthy despite this alarming trend. By incorporating the basic rules outlined in this book into your lifestyle, you can help protect yourself and your loved ones from diabetes and other blood sugar disorders.

HYPOGLYCEMIA

Hypoglycemia, also known as hyperinsulinemia, is the opposite of diabetes because the pancreas secretes *too much* insulin into the bloodstream. When there is too much insulin in the bloodstream, blood sugar levels drop below normal, resulting in glucose starvation at the cellular level, which has a wide variety of negative effects on the body. As with diabetes, the most likely candidates for developing hypoglycemia are those with a family history of the condition and those who undergo prolonged, unresolved stress. The classic signs and symptoms of hypoglycemia (low blood sugar) are:

- Anxiety

- Craving sensations, particularly for alcohol, caffeine, or sweets

- Depression

- Dizziness

- Feeling weak or experiencing a blackout sensation when hungry

- Fatigue or exhaustion

- Headaches
- Inability to concentrate, or "brain fog"
- Insomnia and other sleep disturbances

- Mood swings, emotional upset, and irritability
- Nervousness
- Shakiness

In some individuals, there can be additional symptoms, such as allergies; endocrine disorders (including menstrual irregularity); neurological symptoms such as numbness and tingling; and in some severe cases, fainting or convulsive seizures.

Diagnosing Hypoglycemia

In addition to stress overload and a high dietary intake of refined sugars and starches, a variety of other factors can cause hypoglycemia. These include a reaction to certain drugs such as quinine, some cancers, fever, liver disease, and pregnancy. Sudden drops in blood sugar can also follow very strenuous activity as the body burns glucose for energy.

Laboratory Testing

In conjunction with a comprehensive history and physical examination, the most definitive and accurate means of diagnosing hypoglycemia and diabetes is the six-hour glucose tolerance test. Be aware that most clinics and medical facilities rely on a four-hour glucose tolerance test, which can accurately diagnose full-blown, severe, blood-sugar disorders, but may not be as effective for borderline and milder cases.

Functional Testing

Blood-sugar disturbances are closely linked to stress and the resulting overload and dysfunction of the adrenal glands. Because the adrenal glands cannot work as efficiently, they do not secrete enough anti-insulin hormone. Therefore, levels of insulin in the bloodstream remain high, keeping blood sugar levels low. When I suspect that a patient has low blood sugar, I routinely perform two simple functional tests to learn if the adrenal glands are fatigued and are, therefore, unable to meet the body's needs.

The Light Reflex Pupil Response Test. The light reflex pupil response test is conducted in a darkened examination room. In dim light, the natural response of the iris is to relax, allowing the pupil to widen. To reinforce this relaxation response, the patient is asked to close his or her eyes for a few additional seconds, so that upon reopening the eyes, the pupil will be dilated. Then the doctor shines a small, bright light into the patient's eyes. If the adrenal glands are responding properly, the pupil will immediately become much smaller and, under normal circumstances, the eye remains at that same level of constriction for at least thirty consecutive seconds. If the adrenals are weak or fatigued, however, the pupil cannot maintain steady constriction, and it wavers between constriction and dilation.

The Blood Pressure Test for Adrenal Function. When a doctor or nurse checks a patient's blood pressure, it is traditionally performed with that person either sitting or lying down. However, in the blood pressure test for adrenal exhaustion, the examiner checks and records the blood pressure while the person assumes three different postures. Initially the blood pressure is checked while the patient is lying flat. With the blood pressure cuff still on the patient's arm, she or he is then asked to sit up, and the blood pressure is again checked and recorded. For the third position, the patient is asked to stand up and the examiner evaluates and records the blood pressure a third time. If adrenal function is normal, blood pressure should be slightly higher when the patient sits and stands because more work is required by the heart and blood vessels to move the blood to the various parts of the body than when we are lying down. The extra exertion of the heart and blood vessels is recorded as blood pressure. If the patient's blood pressure does not go up slightly with each change of posture or, as we often find, blood pressure actually drops instead of rising, there is a good chance that the adrenal glands are incapable of adequately responding to the body's work and activity needs.

Clinical Management of Hypoglycemia

Scientists recently confirmed what many have believed for centuries, that there is a direct relationship between blood-sugar levels and anxiety, depressed moods, full-blown clinical depression, negative attitudes, and stress. Stress reduction and improved stress management can almost immediately improve blood-sugar levels and symptoms of blood-sugar disorders. People feel and function better because they have healthy levels of the necessary adrenocortical hormones—secreted by the adrenal glands—in their blood. Because stress management remains one of the greatest challenges in our hectic world, it is important to understand other powerful ways to balance blood-sugar levels. Effectively dealing with these emotional and spiritual factors can be very worthwhile.

Nutritional intervention is an excellent place to start addressing this complex family of disorders. Supplementing with the right nutrients, such as the trace mineral chromium, can be a valuable strategy in the management of blood-sugar disorders. In terms of diet, the most effective means of preventing and managing hypoglycemia is to reduce your intake of alcohol, caffeine, refined starches, and sugars so that the pancreas is not overworked. It is highly rewarding when people find that, by carefully following the required dietary and nutritional discipline, their mood and attitude often improve dramatically.

Therefore, from a natural health standpoint, and with due consideration for individuality and severity of symptoms, I initially give my patients a sheet listing the twelve most common symptoms. They are asked to indicate the presence and severity of their symptoms by using one x for mild, two (xx) for moderate, three (xxx) if more severe, and four (xxxx) for extreme symptoms that could even be partially disabling. If their responses are positive for eight or more symptoms on the list, and their severity indications average more than mild, I suggest the following.

Consume as Much as Desired

- Almost all raw fresh fruits and vegetables

- A wide selection of fish and sea foods

- Caffeine-free herbal teas

- Fresh organic carrot juice

- Raw, fresh nuts and seeds

- Whole grain cereals and breads

- Yogurt (plain, unsweetened)

Permitted in Moderation

- All fruit juices, except grape and prune juices

- Certified raw cow or goat milk

- Chicken, turkey, goose, lamb, and veal

- Dried fruits and dates

- Honey or maple syrup as a sweetener

- Molasses

- Most fruits and vegetables (fresh, raw, cooked, frozen, or canned)

- Mushrooms

- Natural vegetable/mineral seasonings

- Natural plant oils, such as extra virgin olive, flax, sesame, safflower, and primrose oils

- Sweet cream butter

- Unpolished rice

Avoid Totally

- All forms of alcohol

- Bananas, dates, figs, potatoes, white rice, and raisins

- Products containing caffeine, such as chocolate, coffee, colas, and tea

- Many over-the-counter pain relievers such as Anacin and Excedrin, as these products also contain caffeine and temporarily elevate the blood sugar and aggravate the condition in the long run

- Pastas

- Refined cane and beet sugar products, including baked desserts, candy, catsup, corn syrup, custards, ice cream, jams and jellies, Jell-O, pudding, sodas (including diet sodas), and whipped cream

- Sugar substitutes and artificial sweeteners such as aspartame

In addition, it is important to keep the body chemistry alkaline by following the dietary information provided in Chapter 4. And remember that a balanced, regular exercise program can be extremely effective in stabilizing blood-sugar disorders.

THYROID GLAND FACTORS

Anyone struggling with the symptoms of a blood-sugar disorder should also be aware that thyroid gland imbalances can mimic sugar metabolism conditions. Arthritis, depression, fatigue, high cholesterol, infertility, low sex drive, overweight, skin conditions, and other troublesome symptoms can all result from problems with the thyroid gland. Since the health of the endocrine system depends upon a balance of all glandular activity, thyroid conditions can also play a role in poor pancreatic and adrenal functioning. For more information on this topic and practical ways to enhance thyroid function, I recommend *Thyroid Power—10 Steps to Total Health* by Richard L. Shames, M.D., and Karilee Halo Shames, R.N., Ph.D.

SUMMARY

People with diabetes and other blood-sugar disorders who faithfully follow the dietary program outlined in this book, adopt a reasonable exercise program, and take active steps to reduce and manage the stresses in their life can be almost guaranteed to feel better than they have in years. In fact, for some people, following the Golden Rules can minimize the amount of insulin they need. Adopting a healthy diet, supplementation, and exercise program can also greatly reduce the symptoms and risks of non-insulin-dependent diabetes. Avoiding alcohol, caffeine, nicotine, refined starches, soft drinks, and sweets—all acid-forming foods and substances—goes a long way in controlling the symptoms of hypoglycemia and greatly reduces the chances for diabetic complications. Eating small meals and eating more frequently, about every two or three hours, is also an important strategy in controlling blood sugar levels. By selecting a clinician who truly understands the development and treatment of blood-sugar disorders, you can expect to see improvement in your condition. If you fail to notice any improvement after having followed this program for two or three months, you may need further testing to see if a different condition is causing symptoms similar to those known in blood sugar disorders.

13. Headaches

I't's estimated that one out of every five Americans uses pain-relieving drugs daily for the management of headaches. Headaches can have many different causes. If you experience severe, recurrent headaches, it's very important to schedule an appointment with your doctor so you can get an accurate diagnosis to rule out a more serious condition such as a brain tumor, a weakened blood vessel, an infection, or high blood pressure. Once these conditions have been ruled out and your doctor has determined the probable source of your headaches, you can explore appropriate treatment options.

TYPES OF HEADACHES

To weigh your treatment options, it may be helpful to understand exactly what type of headaches you have. The following are the principal types of headaches.

Tension Headache

Tension headaches, in which pain is experienced through the back of the skull, the forehead, and above the eyes, are perhaps the most common type of headache. People who experience tension headaches often complain of accompanying stiffness, fatigue, and tightness in the neck and upper spine, which is usually caused by the muscles in the neck, shoulders, and upper-back being tightly contracted. In fact, tension headaches are often referred to as muscle-contraction headaches.

While the pain of a tension headache can sometimes be severe, tension headaches more often cause moderate pain and are generally not disabling. However, tension headaches tend to be chronic and can negatively affect the enjoyment and quality of everyday activities. Tension headaches are generally experienced by people who are fearful or anxious and have difficulty managing stress in their lives. They are also more common in individuals with unresolved emotional issues who have difficulty relaxing or do not get enough sustained, deep sleep. However, physical factors have also been linked to the frequent onset of tension headaches. For example, previous injuries of the neck and upper spine, as well as long-standing fatigue, constipation, and general states of toxicity must also be considered in understanding and managing tension headaches.

Migraine Headache

Currently, in the United States, approximately 18 percent of women and 6 percent of men experience migraines, which cause severe pain, predominantly on one side of the head, from the back of the skull to the eye and the tissues around the eye. The pain is often intense and throbbing, even causing temporary disability that requires rest in a dark, quiet room until the attack subsides. In addition, most people experience one or more of the following symptoms: anxiety, depression, nausea, weakness and dizziness, sensitivity to noise and light, tingling in the extremities, visual disturbances such as flashing lights, and vomiting. Some people may also experience agitation, diarrhea, disorientation, frequent urination, and tingling on the top of their head along the scalp. In rare cases, a migraine attack can result in temporary paralysis of half of the entire body. Many who suffer from migraines describe an aura, light flashes, visual spots, zigzag lines, or sensitivity to lights and sounds, or experience a feeling of fatigue and sluggishness prior to the actual onset of the pain. Women who get migraines often experience these headaches prior to, or during, their menstrual period.

Many experts speculate that there may be a strong genetic predisposition to migraines. Additionally, some foods are known to trigger migraines, including foods that contain tyramine, such as aged cheeses, bananas, certain nuts, pork, shellfish, and red wine.

The following recommendations can help reduce the frequency and severity of migraines:

- Avoid foods that are known to trigger migraines, including artificial sweeteners such as aspartame, which are contained in all diet sodas and some sugar-free foods; caffeine and caffeine products; and monosodium glutamate (MSG).

- Learn to better manage stress in your life by using stress-reduction and relaxation techniques, such as biofeedback, color therapies, meditation, music, visual imagery, and yoga.

- Consider the use of acupuncture, traditional Chinese medicine, aromatherapy, and massage therapy.

- Feverfew is an herb that can greatly assist in the prevention of migraines.

- Incorporate exercise and stretching into your daily routine.

- Let go of anger, resentment, distrust, and bitterness. Live your faith.

- If you experience frequent and long-standing constipation, seek treatment to alleviate the problem.

- Because migraine is an acid condition, keep your body chemistry alkaline.

- Make sure you get plenty of rest and natural, uninterrupted sleep.

- If you are a perfectionist, try not to be too hard on yourself. A neurologist friend once told me that he had never treated a migraine patient who could go to sleep knowing they had left a sink full of dirty dishes.

- Schedule an appointment with a chiropractor for a thorough, comprehensive evaluation of your structural frame. Countless people with migraine headaches have experienced complete resolution of their disorder from careful, competent chiropractic or other forms of structural care.

- Electro-dermal screening (EDS) can be very useful in pinpointing unexplained sources of energy imbalance, environmental allergies, food, heavy metal or chemical toxicity, or microbial infestation. (See Chapter 9 for more information on this important topic.)

Temporomandibular Joint (TMJ) Disorder Headaches

If your headaches are in the region of your temples, jaw and cheek muscles, ears, eye region, face, neck, and shoulder areas, you may have a condition known as temporomandibular joint (TMJ) disorder. TMJ disorder can cause severe headaches, as well as a long list of other health disorders. Grating, popping, snapping, or tenderness in the jaw joints indicate that there is a structural problem, such as an overbite or some malocclusion of the teeth. TMJ headaches can also result from structural disorders of the neck joints. For this reason, some people may experience TMJ headaches following whiplash trauma to the neck resulting from an accident, or from being struck in the face with an airbag after a head-on automobile collision. Missing teeth, particularly in the lower jaw near the back of the mouth, can also cause TMJ disorders because there is not adequate vertical support for the jaw mechanism. Likewise, people who grind their teeth during sleep are at greater risk of developing TMJ and the accompanying headaches.

If you feel that you may be experiencing symptoms of TMJ disorder, consult a holistically trained dentist who clearly understands this complex problem. It can change your life. In addition, because the jaw joints and the upper spine and neck are the areas usually affected in TMJ disorders, you might want to try acupuncture, aromatherapy, chiropractic, herbal therapies, massage, physical therapy, or stress-reduction techniques to find long-term relief from this disorder.

Cluster Headaches (Horton's Syndrome)

Cluster headaches have a very clear pattern and are reasonably easy to diagnose, as they are distinguished by an extremely intense, one-sided head and facial pain that seems to be concentrated in or behind one eye. Men are more likely to experience cluster headaches than women. Unlike migraine attacks, cluster headaches usually resolve in one to three hours, only to return a few hours later. Although the patterns vary, this type of headache generally comes on in clusters that can last for days or weeks, followed by weeks or months of total relief. Because cluster headaches are often accompanied by congestion that includes nasal secretions, and the eye on the painful side may be watery, people who suffer these headaches may believe they have a sinus infection. Bright sunshine may trigger or aggravate cluster headaches, and a strong link has also been established between alcohol abuse and this type of headache.

Sinus Headaches

The sinuses can also be a source of severe headache pain. Sinus cavities within the skull serve a variety of functions, including cleansing and warming the air you breathe before it enters your lungs. Healthy sinuses also give resonance to your voice and assist your balance and hearing.

Headache pain can result from a variety of sinus problems, including inflammation and infection from bacteria, viruses, or other microbes; injury from external blows in sports or automobile accidents; and polyps in the sinus cavities from allergies or other irritants to the mucous membranes that line these sensitive tissues. In some cases, the nerves that supply the sinus cavities can become inflamed, causing severe head and facial pain.

If you experience prolonged and resistant headaches, it is a good idea to determine the actual cause of your sinus condition—a process that may take some time and sophisticated testing. Once the cause of your sinus problems and related headaches has been established, appropriate treatment can bring about remarkable relief, and even full recovery.

Cervicogenic Headaches

In the past several years, scientific evidence has linked headaches to mechanical disturbances in the joints and related soft-tissue support system of the neck and upper spine. Until recently, these types of headaches, called cervicogenic headaches, were considered difficult to treat. However, we now know that cervicogenic headaches respond very well to hands-on care—chiropractic, osteopathic, physical, or occupational therapy, for example—that improves joint function and relieves inflamed nerves, blood vessels, muscles, and soft tissues. Specific stretching exercises, stress-management techniques, dietary changes, and nutritional supplementation can also be very helpful in alleviating headaches caused by poor joint health and muscle strain in the neck and upper back.

Rebound Headaches

Are you taking too much or too many pain relievers to get rid of your headaches? Rebound headaches can result from taking too much pain medication, even over-the-counter products. Similarly, if you habitually drink caffeinated beverages and you suddenly stop drinking your morning coffee or afternoon sodas, you may also suffer from rebound headaches.

Other Factors in Headache Pain

The causes of headaches are numerous, and include not only those factors listed above, but also health concerns such as chemical exposure, constipation, fluid retention, food and environmental allergies, hormonal imbalance, low blood sugar, poor eyesight, buildup of toxic waste products, and use of birth control pills. If you feel that toxicity may be causing your headaches, you might want to consider having a liver and gallbladder flush, which can effectively reduce general body toxicity, and at the same time soften and flush out small gallstones. Some people have also reported great improvement in problems such as bloating, indigestion, and heartburn after this simple and inexpensive detoxifying process. Ask your holistic healthcare practitioner for specific information about the procedure.

ICE OR HEAT TO RELIEVE HEADACHE PAIN?

Most headache pain originates from blood vessels of the scalp and face that are either excessively dilated or excessively constricted. For headaches that are due to dilated blood vessels, causing a throbbing feeling with every heartbeat, using an ice pack can be very beneficial in relieving the pain. On the other hand, constant headaches that do not have this throbbing pain are due to the constriction of blood vessels and it's best to use moist heat on the back of the head and neck muscles to alleviate these types of headaches. A hot shower followed by a soothing massage also work wonders if you are seeking relief from headaches caused by blood-vessel constriction.

NUTRIENTS FOR HEADACHE PREVENTION

By now, it shouldn't surprise you to know that specific nutrients can be very helpful in preventing the onset of headaches. For example, the common B vitamin niacin can be safely used to gently dilate constricted blood vessels and help relieve pain. Be aware, however, that niacin taken in doses of more than 100 mg can cause a harmless, temporary flushing of the skin. Peppermint, rosemary, and sage are herbal remedies that have been used successfully in managing headaches. Because stress reduction is of great importance for people with headaches, the minerals calcium and magnesium and the herb valerian root can be very beneficial in relaxing muscles, soothing nerves, and promoting sleep. Supplementation with vitamin B$_6$ and zinc has been proven valuable in preventing and managing cluster headaches, while stabilizing blood sugar levels with a balanced diet. Appropriate supplementation is also useful in managing hypoglycemic headaches. (See Chapter 12 for a discussion of hypoglycemia.)

WHEN TO CONSULT A NEUROLOGIST

If you are continuously bothered by severe headaches that seem never to go away, you may need to consult a neurologist who may accurately pinpoint the source of the problem. There are board-certified neurologists in general medicine, chiropractic, and osteopathy who have the research and resources available to correctly diagnose the cause of headache pain.

For many people, chronic headaches cause more than pain—they also cause years of stress spent worrying that a brain tumor or some other life-threatening condition is causing their headaches. Worse still, the resulting anxiety associated with these thoughts can keep the pain cycle active. It is not uncommon for neurologists to order special tests and diagnostic images in order to arrive at a correct diagnosis. If you are worried about the source of your chronic headaches, you may wish to speak to a neurologist about some important tests that can ease your mind.

While it is, of course, advisable to consult a neurologist if you suffer any type of recurring headaches, certain symptoms are sometimes considered to be red flags of more serious conditions and certainly warrant prompt attention. These include sudden, severe pain that occurs with confusion, drowsiness, fever, nausea, stiff neck, or vomiting; any headache that produces a change from usual behavior, confusion, generalized weakness, numbness, slurred speech, or visual disturbances; any headache that is accompanied by a convulsive seizure; and any headache that is the result of a direct blow to the head or a fall onto the head or neck.

NATURAL APPROACHES TO TREATING HEADACHES

Just as fatigue is not likely the result of a lack of caffeine in the body, headaches are not likely the result of a deficiency of aspirin—or other pain medications—in the bloodstream. The truth of the matter is that more than 90 percent of headaches, regardless of their classification, can be treated with great success with one or more natural, drug-free approaches.

For a comprehensive overview of different varieties of headaches, their causes, and a balanced and practical alternative approach to their management, I recommend *An Alternative Medicine Definitive Guide to Headaches* by Burton Goldberg, Robert Milne, M.D., and Blake More.

14. Managing Your Weight

Are you a lean, mean loving machine with buns of steel and sex appeal? It is estimated that up to 70 percent of Americans are overweight. Of this number, about 10 percent are considered obese, and their excess weight is actually threatening their lives. Clearly, for good health, it's important to maintain your weight within a reasonable range.

Many factors need to be considered in understanding the causes of obesity. During the past decade, thousands of low-fat and non-fat products have become available to millions of consumers. You may be surprised to learn that the American Heart Association has pinpointed these products as being major factors in increasing, rather than decreasing, our country's obesity epidemic. How is this possible? Too often, people believe that they can gorge themselves on low-fat cookies, frozen yogurt, ice cream, and pastries. As it turns out, while lower in fat, almost all of these foods contain more sugar and more calories than the full-fat foods.

When you've stopped off at the shopping mall, or any other popular spots that's often crowded with people, have you noticed that the great majority of people who are limping or using canes are significantly overweight? During a recent public radio program focusing on America's image to people living outside the United States, one of the callers who had recently visited America said he was struck by the fact that, in America, "Even the poor people are fat."

EAT, DRINK, AND BE MERRY

The primary reason obesity is so widespread in the United States is poor dietary habits. Occasionally, glandular conditions, such as thyroid disorders, may be the underlying cause of excess weight, but this is quite rare, and treatable once a correct diagnosis is made. Additionally, in women past the age of thirty-five, it's common to be estrogen-dominant, which can result in fluid retention, weight gain, and a variety of other symptoms that relate to menopausal-related hormonal imbalance issues. (See Chapter 6.)

In some cases, genetics is actually at the root of excess weight and obesity—you may, in fact, have inherited a tendency to be overweight. But your genes aren't all that come from your family. You may also have developed many of the same food selection, eating, and cooking habits as your grandparents, parents, brothers and sisters, as well as many of their attitudes about self-esteem and other beliefs about health and health maintenance. For this reason, it's critical to take an active, responsible approach to managing your health and preventing many diseases that can develop as a result of being overweight.

WEIGHT-LOSS PROGRAMS

It may interest you to know that Americans spend over $90 billion annually in weight-loss products and supervised, personalized weight-loss programs offered by professional clinics throughout the country. Of course, all of these corporations claim extraordinary success with their clients; however, what the public does not know is that over 90 percent of all those who lose more than fifty pounds through participation in these programs regain the weight they lost within five years. When surveys were conducted among the 10 percent who were able to keep off the weight, an interesting pattern emerged. This 10 percent did more than restrict and modify their diet and exercise programs—they often reported that they had successfully addressed major self-destructive, stressful behavior patterns in their lives. For this successful 10 percent, there was a realization that their overeating was symptomatic of a deeper, long-term self-image disorder. Eating had become a form of addiction that had to be overcome through participation in self-help and support groups, counseling, meditation, and other stress-reduction programs. In essence, they had to learn to care enough about themselves to change their self-destructive, compulsive behavior patterns.

OBESITY IN CHILDREN

In January of 2002, the U.S. Surgeon General officially declared childhood obesity a national epidemic. Why are so many of America's children struggling with excess weight? One major factor is the approximately 12 billion dollars spent each year on advertising targeted mainly at children. Among the most popular products marketed to young people are high-calorie fast foods, sweets, sodas, Ho-Ho's, Twinkies, sweetened cereals, and other unhealthy foods. McDonald's alone spends over a billion dollars each year for their "Big Mac with Cheese,

French Fries, and a Shake" message. The result of this disregard for the health and wellness of our future generations is plain for all to see in the number of obese or grossly overweight children, which has doubled over the past twenty years. According to the Centers for Disease Control, hospital-related costs for childhood obesity have more than tripled during this time, and black and Hispanic children are particularly at risk.

Obesity among young people is one of the most troubling social concerns of this century, particularly because of its many related health concerns, from diabetes and cancer to high cholesterol, heart disease, and hypertension. Children spend an average of eight hours a day watching television or playing video games, and the profit-driven corporate food giants take full advantage of this highly impressionable age group that has such a huge influence on food purchases in this country.

Calling a Spade a Spade

For the above reasons, Norway and Sweden have already banned junk food advertising to children. (Recent reports indicate that the dietary habits of Europeans are now more like those of Americans, with the same negative health consequences.) Unfortunately, the United States has no similar plans. Just look at how we had to struggle for over forty years to prohibit advertisements for tobacco and nicotine products from being aired, despite the fact that diseases related to the use of these products had been recognized for decades prior to this legislation. While I am a strong supporter of free enterprise and a free economy, I believe that socially minded citizens must act on available information about junk foods and other products known to represent a serious threat to the well-being and health of our nation. For a well-researched and enlightening exploration into the nether world of the fast-foods industry, I urge you to read *Fast Food Nation* by Eric Schlosser. This information will help you understand why the so-called bargain menus offered at fast food restaurants aren't such a bargain when you weigh those dollars against the money spent treating conditions related to obesity.

What Can You Do?

As with many other problems that are widespread throughout our society, the most effective solution to the obesity epidemic in the United States is found at home. Common sense would tell you that allowing a child to play in an area infested with rattlesnakes or black widow spiders is not acceptable, even to the most liberal parents. No thoughtful parent feeds their children whiskey or allows them to use chewing tobacco. Similarly, high-fat foods loaded with refined sugar and salt represent threats of an almost equal magnitude. Parents make the decisions about which foods, snacks, and beverages they buy for their families. They prepare and serve the foods, and therefore, have control of their children's diet and food selection, at least until their children reach school age and are exposed to other dietary choices, by which time food habits are generally established.

Teach by example. Parents are their child's first, most significant teacher for all the important aspects of balanced living. The combination of readily available quantities of candy, cookies, fast foods, presweetened cereals, and sodas, and the excessive amount of time spent watching television and playing video games rather than getting fresh air and exercise sets the stage for a lifetime of obesity and the diseases that are the natural consequence of this type of lifestyle.

Raising and caring for healthy children can be a challenge but, fortunately, the fun and joyful times greatly outweigh the associated stresses. On the other hand, raising and caring for chronically ill children can be a very difficult and stressful experience. Parents, please realize health disorders in children are often related to poor nutrition. Do your homework and learn how to watch what your children eat and guide them in making healthful choices. Don't be afraid to supplement your children's diet with appropriate vitamin and mineral supplements—their lives may depend on it. Growing children are often deficient in some of the nutrients required for health, many of which are not available in adequate amounts in the standard American diet (SAD).

A recent study in Finland showed that infants given 2,000 IU (international units) of vitamin D daily were found to have an 80-percent less chance of developing type I diabetes over the next thirty years than those receiving a smaller dose. People living in Finland are exposed to less sunlight than people living in other areas of the world, and because sunlight is a major factor in the body's manufacture of vitamin D, these findings may not be as relevant for children who live in climates where there is more exposure to sunlight. But this study serves as an example of the potential benefits of improved nutrition for children and adults of all ages.

Self-Esteem

Learning to love oneself is not always easy in a culture that has somehow equated doing so with vanity, conceit, arrogance, and pride. Children who grow up with a self-defeating attitude because they may have been deprived of adequate nurturing, praise, and affection are particularly at risk for developing serious problems with self-image as adults. Loving yourself enough to be able to enjoy the life you deserve should be your life goal. It's not vain to do so—in fact, it's quite the opposite. A person with an alcohol or drug addiction who makes the decision to get clean and sober isn't doing so out of vanity. That person is choosing to change his or her life in order to save it. Such a conscious act of self-love results from the persistent, urgent nurturing of the soul.

If you have struggled with your weight continuously throughout your life, you may wish to seek solutions that include a practical, holistic approach to your needs from a physical, emotional, and spiritual perspective. An excellent, highly respected organization known as TOPS (Take Off Pounds Sensibly), which embraces the holistic philosophy of weight management, has helped millions of people who were once overweight positively change their lives in profound ways. For more information, you can call 1-800-932-8677 or visit their website at www.TOPS.org.

Nutritional Supplementation May Help

Certain nutritional supplements may also be effective in suppressing appetite and helping to change eating behaviors. For instance, the serotonin supplement 5-HTP, although somewhat expensive, has been proven safe and works for 70 to 80 percent of people who use it. It is also effective for overweight people with type I or type II diabetes, and especially those who crave sweets and refined starch foods. People who are trying to manage blood sugar disorders ranging from hypoglycemia to diabetes may wish to plan meals and snacks using the glycemic index, which rates foods containing sugars and starches in proportion to their potential effect on blood sugar levels.

An excellent overview of the psychological and physiological issues tied to overeating are provided in Chris Fairburn's excellent books *Overcoming Binge Eating* and, coauthored with Kelly Brownell, *Eating Disorders and Obesity: A Comprehensive Handbook*. Also, *Inspired to Lose* by Dr. Howard Rankin is a highly motivational book for those struggling with weight concerns. The guiding principles expressed in these works are at once refreshing and practical. You can also learn more about the causes and consequences of dangerous dietary habits by contacting Overeaters Anonymous at www.overeatersanonymous.org or the National Eating Disorders Association at www.nationaleatingdisorders.org.

Anorexia and Bulimia

Young people often struggle with body image and become psychologically and physically obsessive about weight and its relationship to their appearance and social acceptance. Therefore, any discussion on weight management would not be complete without briefly addressing two very serious health conditions, anorexia nervosa and bulimia nervosa. If you or someone you love is struggling with anorexia or bulimia, a holistic approach to treatment may be beneficial because almost no clinical disorder has a more clearly defined relationship among body, mind, and spirit.

Anorexia nervosa is identified by prolonged avoidance of eating, with a total aversion to food for fear of becoming fat. Unrealistic identification with popular movie stars and music idols often serves as the catalyst for the food aversion, malnutrition, and eventual starvation that are the hallmarks of this heartbreaking disorder. Bulimia nervosa is characterized by binge eating followed by self-induced vomiting, or the use of diuretics and laxatives to maintain what the person perceives to be a normal weight. Both anorexia and bulimia must be considered forms of gradual suicide.

In recent years, more attention has been focused on the grave consequences of both anorexia and bulimia, especially in younger females, although a rise in both disorders has recently been noted among older women, as well. It's estimated that as many as 20 percent of college women engage in mild or moderate forms of bulimic behaviors. Family members, friends, and caregivers of people who have eating disorders, as well as the people struggling with these conditions themselves, must all take the occurrence of anorexia and bulimia very seriously. In almost all cases, professional help is required. For further information, contact the National Association of Anorexia Nervosa and Associated Disorders at www.anad.org. It is the nation's oldest national nonprofit organization for helping people with eating disorders and their families. I also recommend reading the very inspirational book *Anorexia Nervosa: A Guide to Recovery* by Lindsey Hale and Martha Ostroff.

Finally, by now you should not be surprised to learn that a natural result of simply following the Golden Rules for good health will be the realization of the right body weight for your frame. Can it really be that simple? Yes, it can.

15. Arthritis

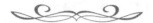

Jf you have arthritis in any of its forms, carefully following the advice provided in this chapter and throughout the book can help you overcome many of its effects. If your arthritis is advanced, severe, and notably disabling, you may wish to explore safe, natural substances that have been proven beneficial in alleviating the pain, stiffness, and other symptoms associated with the many forms of this condition. Initially, however, it may be useful to review the most common types of arthritis in order to choose the most effective natural-control measures available.

TYPES OF ARTHRITIS

Osteoarthritis

Approximately 40 million people in the United States are living with osteoarthritis, or degenerative joint disease, a painful and often disabling condition. By degenerative, we mean that the disease worsens with age. While almost all joints in the body are affected by this condition, the greatest amount of degeneration occurs in the weight-bearing joints, such as the lower spine, hips, knees, and ankles. It can also cause disfiguring and painful destruction of the hand and shoulder joints. Osteoarthritis is a major source of chronic disability, leading to a diminished quality of life, lost wages and work productivity, and enormous medical expense.

In addition to the wear-and-tear effects of the aging process, another source of joint destruction occurs that is secondary to trauma. Traumatic injury to joints from athletic activities and automotive or industrial accidents often results in the early breakdown and destruction of cartilage, the firm, dense, gelatin-based tissue within joints that absorbs shock and facilitates smooth, quiet, friction-free motion. Most joints are also bathed in a lubricating liquid called synovial fluid, which is contained in a dense, thin membrane known as the joint capsule. Arthritis, literally translated as "joint inflammation," results when the cartilage and surrounding joint capsule are damaged or wear thin.

Arthritis symptoms usually progress very slowly and include low-grade swelling, stiffness, and pain. As joint health continues to deteriorate, creaking, popping, and grinding sounds are felt and heard within the affected joints. Stiffness in the joints is usually most pronounced in the morning after sleep, or after prolonged sitting or other inactivity during the day, but improves with movement. However, if work or recreational activity is too intense pain and swelling return, and only rest can provide at least temporary relief.

People who have severe, advanced, degenerative arthritis often undergo a total surgical joint replacement. If the pain of arthritis cannot be managed or alleviated, surgeons must fuse the surfaces of the joints together using screws, pins, wire, or other metallic stabilizers to prevent motion within the joint. Although this procedure usually offers total pain relief, there is no movement in the joint after the surgery.

Adult Rheumatoid Arthritis

Adult rheumatoid arthritis most commonly occurs in people between twenty and forty years of age. This deforming, degenerative disease usually affects the joints of the hands, wrists, elbows, shoulders, ankles, feet, and knees. The cause of rheumatoid arthritis is as yet unknown and the condition is difficult to treat. Initially, the symptoms of the disease include pain, swelling, and stiffness of the joints, which is most pronounced in the mornings upon awakening. Gradually, the joints become more tender and the muscles around the joints become spastic. In time, reluctance to move the joints due to severe pain results in muscle wasting, and the surrounding muscles are weakened and shrink from lack of use. After the disease has run its course, which may take up to twenty or more years, about 50 percent of those who have struggled with the condition recover enough to go back to their previous occupations. About 10 percent, however, never recover and are severely disabled and confined to bed or a wheelchair. The diagnosis of rheumatoid arthritis is based on the clinical presentation, age, gender, and certain blood tests.

As researchers have learned more about rheumatoid arthritis, it's become clear that certain factors significantly predispose individuals to the disease. According to a study in the *Annals of the Rheumatic Diseases* (2001), the use of hair dyes for more than twenty years increased the risk of rheumatoid arthritis in women 1.9 times; those using insulin replacement therapy for diabetes had a ten-fold rate of the disease; and the psychosocial stress related to marital quarrels resulted in a nine-fold rate, compared to the control group. Other factors that showed an increased rate of the disease in this study were tick-borne infections, exposure to horses, short fertility period, smoking, and previous injury. Also, in men, the use of private well water and exposure to mold indoors were linked to the development of rheumatoid arthritis. Occupational hairdressing has also been linked to the development of rheumatoid arthritis (as well as the blood cancer known as lymphoma). Clearly, because we do understand some of the predispositions to rheumatoid arthritis, it's possible to take measures to prevent the development of the condition in some cases.

Juvenile Arthritis

Juvenile arthritis is similar to forms of arthritis that adults suffer in that it affects five or more joints and occasionally other body systems, as well, causing anemia, enlargement of the spleen, fever, swelling in lymph glands, and skin rash. Female children are more likely to develop this condition than are male children. For all children who are affected, however, over 90 percent of the time juvenile arthritis does not develop into adult rheumatoid arthritis.

Ankylosing Spondylitis (AS)

Ankylosing spondylitis (AS) is a form of arthritis that affects the sacroiliac and spinal joints of young adults. AS usually develops in young people in their late teens and is almost never diagnosed in patients after age thirty. Men are somewhat more predisposed to developing the condition. The disease first affects the sacroiliac joints and gradually spreads upward along the spine, causing all the spinal joints to become fused and resulting in spinal stiffness and rigidity. Eventually, the spine is pulled into a forward bent posture, in some cases so pronounced that the patient is incapable of looking straight ahead. Even minor trauma can cause spinal fractures and the condition is often accompanied by low grade fever, significant fatigue, and weight loss. Occasionally, AS may also affect one or both hips, which makes walking very difficult and may result in the need for hip replacement surgery.

Gouty Arthritis

Gout is a painful condition affecting the joints of the feet, particularly in the region of the great toe, that typically strikes middle-aged or older men. There is a family history of the disease in about half the cases, and although the actual cause is unknown, acute attacks of gout, which can last from several days to several weeks, are often related to excessive alcohol use or dietary indiscretion. Injury to the affected area and exposure to cold can also trigger an attack. Large, nodular deposits of sodium monourate crystals, also known as uric acid crystals, form in the tissues surrounding the affected joints, causing pain and, over time, chronic inflammation that gradually destroys cartilage. Eventually, the damage resulting from the inflammatory reaction to uric acid crystals can lead to full-blown degenerative joint disease.

Psoriatic Arthritis

About 2 percent of people with the skin condition psoriasis develop an associated form of arthritis that affects many joints of the body, especially those of the hands and feet. Like other forms of arthritis, this condition can be very painful and can lead to joint degeneration and disability in some people.

Septic or Infectious Arthritis

Septic or infectious arthritis sets in when germs penetrate a joint, either from the bloodstream or through a cut, puncture wound, or scrape. Warning signs of this condition are pain in the region of the joint, muscle spasm, and marked tenderness and swelling. Fortunately, immediate treatment can minimize complications such as joint destruction, dislocation, and joint fusion and rigidity. However, infectious arthritis is one form of arthritis that represents a true emergency, as the infection can spread to other areas of the body through the bloodstream, perhaps even resulting in death.

ORTHODOX TREATMENTS

Most people with the various forms of non-infectious arthritis rely upon over-the-counter (OTC) non-steroidal anti-inflammatory drugs (NSAIDS), including acetaminophen (such as Tylenol), aspirin, or ibuprofen (such as Motrin). While these OTC products provide effective relief for many people, prolonged use of such medications can have serious side effects, including congestive heart failure, fluid retention, gastrointestinal ulceration and bleeding, high blood pressure, and kidney damage. Long-term medical treatments with more potent prescription drugs, such as steroids, can have dangerous side effects, as well, including brittle bones, cataracts of the eyes, change in facial characteristics, cartilage degeneration, reduced resistance to infection, diabetes, and high blood pressure. Other prescribed treatments for arthritis are physical therapy activities; weight reduction; application of heat, cold, electricity, or ultrasound; and graded exercises. For advanced stages of the disease, surgery may be considered as an option.

NATURAL REMEDIES

In recent years, several naturally occurring, non-drug products have become readily available that have been proven beneficial for some people with arthritis inflammation. These products include chondroitin sulfate, glucosamine sulfate, MSM (methyl sulfylmethane), and SAMe (S-adenosyl methionine). Devil's claw root, evening primrose oil, feverfew, flax oil, and quercetin have been observed to provide healing effects to inflamed joints, as well. All of these supplements are available at your local health food store without a prescription, and they are considered safe when taken according to the directions on the label. While some of these products are fairly expensive, it's well worth giving such natural therapies a try for at least ninety days. If you choose to try glucosamine and chondroitin, you'll obtain maximum benefits from taking these products in combination. Because the food source for both glucosamine and chondroitin is gelatin, you may wish to purchase Knox Gelatine powder, available in any food store, and mix it into water or juice, salad dressings, smoothies, or soups. Be aware, however, that Jell-O, which contains small amounts of gelatin, also has large amounts of white sugar and artificial colorings and flavorings, and should be avoided if you are seeking to treat your arthritis naturally.

The following herbal products have valuable anti-inflammatory properties and may be very useful in managing certain arthritis conditions:

- Boswellia, from the gum resin of the boswellia tree

- Bromelain, from pineapple and papaya

- Curcumin, from the spice turmeric

- Devil's claw, with the anti-inflammatory agent known as harpogoside

- Ginger root extract, with oleoresins and gingerols

- White willow bark extract, with anti-inflammatory phenolic glycosides

In addition to the above items, ETA, extracted from mussels, is a natural, over-the-counter product that acts as an effective anti-inflammatory agent for both osteoarthritis and rheumatoid arthritis. These nutraceuticals, when taken properly, have saved many people from a lifetime of painful arthritis. However, it's important to note that because various forms of arthritis have different causes, all types of arthritis may not be equally responsive to all of the above substances.

The Arthritis Foundation offers a free guide that includes its evaluation of sixty-seven different substances that can be helpful in treating arthritis. The guide provides information on the use, effectiveness, and possible side effects of these products, as well as other helpful tips for managing arthritis. You can order a copy by calling 1-800-283-7800 or by visiting the Arthritis Foundation's website at www.arthritis.org.

The Arthritis Trust of America is another organization that can provide a wealth of information about management and treatment of arthritis and rheumatoid diseases. For more information, call 1-615-799-1002 or visit the organization's website at www.arthritistrust.org to find useful links and a list of practitioners who can help you find relief from your arthritis.

Myofascial Release Therapy

The fascia is a tough connective-tissue web that envelops all the muscles of the body from head to toe. Fascial restrictions do not show up in traditional medical evaluations, such as x-rays and laboratory tests, so many people are unaware of the profoundly negative impact these adhesions can have on their comfort and well-being. Myofascial release therapy is a gentle, hands-on treatment developed by John Barnes, a physical therapist who has shown notable success using the technique to release adhesions in the fascial system, as well as in other areas of tension or stress. The treatment can provide lasting relief for anyone with aches, pains, and stiffness—including, of course, people with arthritis.

The Graston Technique

Graston instrument technique is a highly effective means of releasing adhesions found in fascia, joint, muscle, and tendons. This new technique is rapidly becoming popular. The treatment is practiced by a variety of professionals, including chiropractors, occupational therapists, and physical therapists. During treatment, carefully designed stainless steel instruments are manually applied to the restricted myofascial areas to bring about pain relief and increased range of motion. Care may also include heat or ice, along with stretching and strengthening exercises. For further information about the technique and providers in your area, contact Graston Technique, a division of Therapy Care Resources, Inc., at 1-866-926-2828, or visit www.grastontechnique.com.

Respondex

In the early 1990s, Dr. Ted Oslay developed a successful method of managing fascia, joint, muscle, and nerve disorders that combines subtle electrical stimulation with manual probes to gently release accumulated toxins in inflamed and overused tissues. The treatment has been shown to relieve a range of disorders of the spine and the extremities, including carpal tunnel syndrome. For additional information and a list of Respondex practitioners, contact the International Academy of Chiropractic Occupational Health Consultants (IACOHC) at 1-507-455-1025 or www.iacohc.com.

STRESS IS A SIGNIFICANT FACTOR IN ARTHRITIS

Another important consideration in all forms of arthritis and joint inflammation is stress. Prolonged states of anger, fear, and anxiety all overload the adrenals, the glands that secrete the powerful anti-inflammatory hormone cortisone. Because cortisone enables the body to protect the cartilage and lubrication system of the joints, and an overload on the adrenals depletes the body's supply of this protective hormone, any prolonged stress can indirectly cause damage to cartilage and joints. In light of these facts, people with arthritis would do well to carefully reassess how they deal with fear, anger, and other negative emotions in their lives. A generous dose of forgiveness that comes from the core of a person's being can offer real hope for alleviating the pain of arthritis.

ADDITIONAL TIPS FOR MANAGING ARTHRITIS

Attaining normal body weight can be a very important component of your arthritis care program. (For more information, refer to the material on weight management in Chapter 14.) Additionally, exercise and stretching programs can be helpful in controlling arthritis symptoms. In particular, swimming is beneficial because it allows for full-body movement without the impact stress of weight-bearing exercises, while at the same time aiding in weight management and muscle-toning. If you are not a swimmer, you can still help your arthritis by participating in aquatherapy or hydrotherapy exercises in the swimming pool. Many communities have supervised hydrotherapy programs designed specifically for senior citizens, since this is the population most affected by the degenerative joint diseases.

Applying heat to stiff and achy muscles and joints, or taking hot showers or whirlpool baths can also provide some relief from arthritis pain, and heated paraffin baths have been shown to benefit people suffering arthritis of the hands and wrists. Topical heat-producing anti-inflammatory ointments, creams, sprays, and lotions can temporarily relieve aching joints. Products containing capsicum (capsaicin), made from chili peppers, are especially effective.

Reducing stress on the joints is very beneficial in helping to alleviate the pain of arthritis. It's wise to avoid activities that require squatting and kneeling, both of which place a great deal of stress on the joints of the lower extremities, as well as the hips, pelvis, and lower spine. Some people with arthritis use an elevated toilet seat to reduce pressure on the lower spine and hips, knees, and ankles while moving up and down from the seated posture. Handrails that are securely and strategically fastened to walls can be a great aid to comfortable movement into and out of the bathtub, up and down steps, and in confined spaces. If the pain and stiffness of arthritis is severe, mechanical supports, such as a cane or walker, are helpful in reducing stress on inflamed, swollen joints so that you can get around more comfortably. And, of course, as you will recall from Chapter 3, proper shoe size is very important in maintaining joint health. If your arthritis prevents you from sleeping soundly, place a small cushion between your knees if you tend to sleep on your side to help reduce pressure on the joints and alleviate pain.

In many cases, acupuncture, acupressure, myofascial trigger point therapy, massage, castor oil packs, muscle stripping, specific chiropractic manual adjustment, and various forms of mobilization and manipulation can all be very helpful in managing arthritis. A holistically oriented healthcare provider can assist you in the application of each of these therapies based on your individual needs. Finally, because arthritis in all its forms is invariably a disease associated with body acidity, I can't emphasize enough the importance of maintaining an alkaline body chemistry. (Refer back to Chapter 4 for a thorough discussion of acid versus alkaline body chemistry.)

16. Cancer— A Modern Plague

```
~~~C~~~
```

ancer continues to be one of mankind's greatest challenges. In spite of the time, talent, and economic and human resources poured into research and treatment, the disease in all of its forms kills about 500,000 Americans each year. It is the single most significant factor in personal bankruptcy, and approximately 60 percent of all healthcare dollars are expended for cancer-related health issues. While great strides have been made in the fight against cancer—including notable advances in the diagnosis and treatment of lymphoma and childhood leukemia—over 1,000,000 new cases are diagnosed every year, and almost all forms of cancer remain stubbornly present in Western society. In fact, some forms of cancer, such as childhood brain tumors, are even increasing in frequency. Clearly, then, prevention is very important.

When we talk about cancer, we're really referring to a family of diseases. Currently, we know of over one hundred forms of the illness, usually referred to by the organs affected—colon cancer, pancreatic cancer, and skin cancer, to name a few of many. Regardless of type, all forms of cancer begin within the cells, the body's basic structural units. Every second of your life, your body cells reproduce and replace themselves. This means that, every few days, the lining of your stomach has been replaced entirely with new cells; every ninety days, all of the body's billions of skin cells and red blood cells have also been replenished. Thus, every few years, almost all of the body's cells are completely replaced with new, healthy cells.

Cell regeneration and growth is normal. However, with cancer, body cells begin to divide uncontrollably, causing the development of abnormal growths called tumors. Benign tumors are typically confined to a particular area of the body and do not spread throughout the rest of the body. Some benign tumors can be dangerous, however. For example, most tumors of the brain and spinal cord are benign, but over time some of these tumors may slowly enlarge and cause major disruption of bodily functions. Once the benign tumors are removed surgically, they usually do not return. Malignant tumors are more dangerous tumors that grow in an uncontrolled manner, often spreading, or metastasizing, from the original site—such as the bones, brain, liver, or lungs—through the blood or lymph circulation to a secondary site. Because malignant cancers can spread to other areas of the body, they are often life-threatening.

WHO IS AT RISK FOR CANCER?

Cancer affects all economic, social, and ethnic groups worldwide, and although the disease can strike anyone at any age, it develops most frequently in middle-aged and older people. While all body tissues and organs are susceptible to the disease, the colon, lungs, skin, stomach, and breasts—primarily in females—are at the greatest risk of being affected by cancer. In order of frequency, the most common cancers in women are cancers of the breast, lung, cervix, ovaries, lymphatic system, blood (leukemia), uterus, bladder, and stomach. The most common cancers that affect men are cancers of the prostate, lung, colon, lymphatic system, blood (leukemia), bladder, kidney, stomach, and pancreas, again in order of frequency. Cancer is not contagious, so you are not at higher risk of developing the illness even if you have direct contact with someone who is in the advanced stages of the disease.

Known High-Risk Factors

The following are considered the most common, high-risk factors for cancer:

- Alcohol abuse
- Tobacco use
- Obesity and poor diet
- Chemical and environmental exposures to carcinogens including asbestos, benzene, cadmium, nickel, radon, uranium, and vinyl chloride, and other toxic substances such as herbicides and pesticides
- Exposure to radiation from x-rays and other sources
- In the case of skin cancer, excessive exposure to sunlight
- Genetics, although it's still unclear whether this is related to inherited genes that predispose individuals to cancer, or whether it reflects similar behaviors, diets, and lifestyle patterns among family members.

Hormone replacement therapy, particularly estrogen in combination with progestin and a synthetic estrogen hormone known as diethylstilbestrol (DES). While DES is no longer used, the children of women who used this product may be at higher risk for cancers of the cervix, uterus, and vagina in women, and underdevelopment or other abnormalities of the testicles among men.

EARLY SIGNS OF CANCER

The National Cancer Institute lists the following symptoms or warning signs as indicative of cancer:

- A chronic cough or hoarse voice

- Any sore that does not heal

- Changes in bowel or urinary bladder habits

- Indigestion or difficulty swallowing

- Obvious changes in a wart or mole on the skin

- The presence of a lump, or a thickening of the breast or other body part

- Unexplained changes in weight

- Unusual bleeding or discharge

DIAGNOSIS

The first step in managing any form of cancer is early and accurate diagnosis. Your doctor may detect signs of cancer during a routine physical exam, or you may wish to schedule a visit if you have noticed any of the warning signs listed above. Your doctor may order specific medical tests to detect or rule out the possibility of cancer, including blood and urine testing; x-rays; a CAT (computerized axial tomography) scan; endoscopy, which uses lights, mirrors, and cameras to obtain a closer look at the affected area; an MRI (magnetic resonance imaging); nuclear medicine (radionuclide scanning); a sonogram or ultrasound; and surgical biopsy, in which suspicious cells are examined under special microscopes.

In cases where a thorough medical exam and appropriate testing yield a diagnosis of cancer, the doctor making the diagnosis will likely have a cancer specialist called an oncologist confirm the results and give an expert opinion. At that point, the team of doctors presents a variety of treatment options and gives a prognosis, or prediction, regarding the outcome of the disease. Doctors must take many factors into account, including type and stage of the disease, plus the patient's age, general health, and lifestyle, to arrive at an accurate prognosis. Because of the grave nature of the disease and the many life-changing measures that must be taken, it's recommended that anyone who has been diagnosed with cancer obtain a second opinion before choosing any treatment option.

TREATMENT OPTIONS IN WESTERN MEDICINE

Conventional Western medicine offers a wide range of treatments for cancer, and the best option for any individual depends upon location, character, and severity of the disease. Surgery and radiation are local treatments that affect only the cancerous tissues and surrounding area, and have been shown to offer some success in treatment when the cancer has not yet spread to other tissues or organs. Chemotherapy, hormone therapy, and biologic therapy are examples of more generalized forms of care that affect all the cells of the body. Because it's difficult to protect healthy cells from the destructive effects of these therapies designed to kill cancerous cells, most people experience some side effects from treatment.

Bone Marrow Transplants and Stem Cells

Particularly in cancers involving blood-forming tissues, bone marrow transplants may be used to treat the illness. Research is still being conducted to examine the efficacy of using stem cells, which are immature blood cells harvested prior to a diagnosis of cancer. These cells then mature into healthy blood cells to help restore the body's immune system, often damaged from radiation and chemotherapy.

The National Cancer Institute

If you would like to learn more about conventional medical treatments for cancer, you can contact the National Cancer Institute (NCI), the principal federal agency (funded by taxpayers) for cancer research. Its mission is "to stimulate and support scientific discovery and its application to achieve a future when all cancers are uncommon and easily treated." The NCI offers a series of booklets and educational materials available from the Cancer Information Service by calling 1-800-422-6237. You can also order materials from NCI's website at www.cancer.gov. The *What You Need to Know About . . .* educational series includes more than 20 publications. Each booklet provides helpful information about a specific type of cancer and its symptoms, diagnosis, treatment, and emotional issues surrounding the illness, plus important questions to ask the doctor.

AN ALTERNATIVE VIEW

Alternative medicine offers a variety of theories and explanations regarding the development and treatment of cancers that differ substantially from the mainstream position expressed by most practitioners of conventional Western medicine. Indeed, alternative medicine publications have presented many individual case studies and accounts of extraordinary recoveries resulting from natural cancer treatments, without the use of drugs, surgery, or radiation therapy. Of course, there continues to be a great deal of controversy and speculation surrounding the efficacy of alternative treatments, and only time will tell which approach— or combination of approaches—is most effective.

CANCER A SYSTEMIC DISEASE

Many alternative practitioners believe cancer is a systemic disease affecting every cell of a person's body, not a localized disease affecting only one body part or organ. And although cancer is one of the most dreaded and misunderstood diseases of our time, experts agree that the cause is depressed immunity. Most alternative health practitioners recognize four principle reasons for the immune system's breakdown:

1. Poor diet, nutritional imbalances, and obesity

2. Emotional stress

3. Environmental pollutants, with resulting toxic effects on the body

4. Lifestyle factors, including smoking, alcohol and drug use, and so forth

Each of the above factors can have an equally negative impact on health, so you would be wise to take stock of your environment, lifestyle, and daily habits and make any necessary adjustments in order to protect yourself against cancer and other illnesses. By paying careful attention to the Golden Rules outlined in this book, you will be avoiding most of the environmental, lifestyle, nutritional, and toxic pitfalls that can depress the immune system.

Emotional Factors in Cancer

The relationship of *emotional stress* to cancer is very important, and there is some evidence that people with cancer often have many similar personality traits. For example, some people who develop cancer may tend to be perfectionists or overachievers, and may be regarded as somewhat stoic and reluctant to share their true emotions and feelings. Although they may be perfectionists, people with these personality traits tend to be self-critical and have doubts about their worthiness, and they are often self-sacrificing, placing the needs of others before their own, at times even neglecting their own emotional and material needs. In fact, some people may equate suffering in silence with strength of character, or further evidence of their own virtuous behavior.

A noted psychiatrist once proclaimed, based on observations from his practice, that cancer may be a "socially acceptable form of suicide." Confirming the clear relationship between the body, mind, and spirit, he determined that fatal cancers were four times more prevalent in his psychiatric practice than in the general population. While it would not be accurate to suggest that the above personality profile fits all cancer patients, understanding the role emotions play in health and disease is becoming of greater interest to more and more researchers worldwide.

Can Beta Glucan Be Part of the Solution to Cancer Prevention?

Beta glucan is a nontoxic immune-system stimulator that's shown promising benefits in the prevention of cancer and certain severe infectious diseases. Derived from yeast, this all-natural food supplement is available in health food stores or through Life Source Basics. To place an order, you can visit the Life Source Basics website at www.lifesourcebasics.com or call toll free: 1-877-346-6863.

SEEK OUT ADDITIONAL INFORMATION

Dr. Rachel Naomi Remen, Director of the Institute for the Study of Health and Illness at Commonweal in Bolinas, CA, is considered a foremost authority on the body/mind/spirit relationship to cancer and many other very serious diseases. To learn more about the physical, psychological, and spiritual links to the development of cancer and its treatment, contact the Institute. (See Resources and Websites on page 237.)

If you or someone you love has cancer or is a cancer survivor, I urge you to read *The Third Opinion* by John Fink. This extraordinary book is loaded with valuable material about causes, prevention, and treatment, and provides resources and first-rate information on alternative clinics and treatment regimens.

Dr. Samuel Epstein's body of work is an excellent source of information on cancer, with particular emphasis on environmental considerations and prevention. His popular book is entitled *The Politics of Cancer Revisited*.

Among the most respected and professionally referenced books on the natural, nontoxic approach to cancer is *An Alternative Medicine Definitive Guide to Cancer,* a 1,100-page book multi-authored by W. John Diamond, M.D., W. Lee Cowden, M.D., and Burton Goldberg.

Two more excellent books on cancer are *The Cure for All Cancers* and *The Cure for All Advanced Cancers* by Hulda Clark, Ph.D., N.D. (New Century Press, 1-800-519-2465). These works provide dozens of well-documented total reversals cures of even the most advanced cancers of all types. Dr. Clark provides detailed, step-by-step explanations and instructions for both patients and caregivers, and while her program requires total discipline, for those who are willing to follow her advice to the letter, she claims an astounding 95-percent cure rate.

17. Constipation

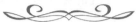

The body's ability to fully eliminate harmful waste products is very important to good health. Through the colon, the organ primarily responsible for detoxification, the body is able to cleanse itself of wastes in order to maintain health. Thus, it's imperative that colon function is effective and efficient. Constipation is a very common disorder among Americans—in fact, Americans spend $450,000,000 annually on commercial laxatives! Fortunately, the Golden Rules presented in this chapter can help you avoid this uncomfortable problem.

ALL CONSTIPATION IS NOT THE SAME

The most common form of constipation is known as atonic constipation, which affects approximately 85 percent of all people who at one time or another must deal with the condition. The less common type of constipation is irritable bowel syndrome (IBS), or spastic constipation. If you regularly suffer constipation, it's important to understand the distinction between the two conditions, because the treatments for each differ significantly.

Atonic Constipation

When the colon wall lacks adequate tone, it is said to be atonic. In atonic constipation, the stool is large, hard, dry, and difficult to pass. For most people, the treatment for this condition is quite simple. The following suggestions can greatly improve the tone of the colon wall to relieve this particular type of constipation:

- Add digestive enzymes to your diet to help your body more completely break down the foods you eat. It's common for older people to have a condition called achlorhydria, in which the body does not produce sufficient amounts of stomach acids to digest food, especially those high in protein such as cheese, eggs, fish, meat, and nuts. Therefore, if you are fifty years of age or older, you may benefit from taking tablets containing a small amount of hydrochloric acid (betaine hydrochloride) with your meals.

- Avoid using diuretics, including alcohol and caffeine products, which dehydrate the body, causing the stool to become dry and hard.

- If you use laxatives, choose only natural, vegetable-based products. Cooked prunes can be beneficial, as well as prune juice, especially if it's warm or heated. Metamucil is an effective natural laxative, and using Necterra Plus regularly can be very helpful in preventing constipation.

- Do not use enemas frequently. Over time, the body develops a dependency on this artificial mechanical stimulation normally provided by nerve and muscle activity.

- Chew your foods thoroughly to aid digestion.

- When nature calls, it is best to heed the signal. If bowel movements are too frequently postponed until a more convenient time, the nerves that regulate the colon become deconditioned.

- Drink more pure water and fresh, raw fruit and vegetable juices.

- Eat more fresh, raw fruits, vegetables, whole grains and high-fiber foods. Organically grown fruit and nut smoothies are excellent for relieving and preventing constipation, and are nourishing, as well.

- Exercise on a regular basis.

- Include more potassium-rich foods in your diet, such as baked beans, bananas, orange juice, oranges, prunes, sweet corn, and spinach.

- Have your spine evaluated for disturbances to the nerves that regulate your colon.

- Occasionally, for severe, long-standing, and resistant atonic constipation, the use of glycerin suppositories, inserted rectally, can be helpful. However, as with enemas, suppositories should not be used too frequently, because of possible deconditioning of the nerves that regulate the colon.

- The stool-softener Colace is available over-the-counter and is safe to use as often as needed.

- While lying on your back with both knees bent, gently but firmly massage and knead the left lower portion of your colon through your abdominal wall.

It is common to find tight, tender areas indicating congestion and compaction of stool. For your comfort, you should empty your urinary bladder before beginning this type of abdominal massage.

It's important to note that taking inorganic iron supplements can cause constipation as a side effect. To maintain or regain optimal blood hemoglobin, it is better to rely on foods rich in organic iron, such as beets, dates, figs, molasses, raisins, spinach, or other dark green vegetables. At one time, mineral oil was recommended to treat constipation, but this is a petroleum-based product that cannot be absorbed by the body and is best avoided.

Spastic Constipation or Irritable Bowel Syndrome (IBS)

Spastic colon, also known as irritable bowel syndrome or IBS, results when the colon wall is constricted and is therefore in a state of low-grade spasm. In cases of IBS, stools are thin, small, and ribbon or pencil-shaped, but may at times be small, round, and hard, resembling marbles. The size and shape of the stools are indications of the constriction of the bowel. If IBS is allowed to progress without treatment, the stools may eventually contain blood, mucus, or both. Therefore, prompt diagnosis and proper treatment is essential.

Management of Spastic Constipation

If you are experiencing spastic constipation, it's important to know that food roughage, laxatives, stimulating high-fiber diets, and spicy foods can aggravate the condition. Therefore, during the initial weeks of care and until the colon wall regains a more normal tone, it's best to stick to a bland diet that includes low-fiber, seed-free cooked vegetables—beans, carrots, peas, potatoes, pumpkin, squash, turnips, and yams, to name a few—as well as cooked or canned fruits. You may also wish to include cream soups, custards, non-sweetened gelatin desserts, pudding, and dairy products (in moderate amounts) in your diet. As with prevention and treatment of atonic constipation, be sure to chew your foods thoroughly to aid digestion. Also, eliminate alcohol, caffeine, and nicotine from your lifestyle, and cut back on your use of spicy seasonings. As the shape, size, and character of the stools begin to normalize, you can gradually return to eating a more traditional balanced and nourishing diet.

Take a Stress Inventory

More than any other body system, the colon mirrors our underlying emotional state, so it's no surprise that terms such as anal retentive, tight ass, and uptight often do approximate the personalities of people with rigid, unyielding attitudes and belief systems. In my experience, people with spastic constipation tend to have unresolved stress in their personal lives; therefore stress management is a key to satisfactory treatment of the disorder.

If you wish to better manage IBS, you may benefit from taking a careful inventory of the various day-to-day stresses you experience, with particular emphasis on relationship issues. An inability to let go and the need to hold on to attitudes, grudges, memories, and regrets from the past are often manifested as disorders of the colon, as are feelings and emotions such as bitterness, fear, guilt, hostility, jealousy, and resentment. These factors must be addressed if you expect to make a full recovery from this challenging condition. Extending forgiveness to those who have hurt you, as well as forgiving yourself for your own indiscretions and inadequacies is an excellent place to begin.

There is some evidence that hypnotherapy, acupressure, acupuncture, chiropractic, and massage can help calm the overactive nerves regulating the colon, thereby aiding in recovery from spastic constipation. More than anything, this shows the importance of a healthy body/mind/spirit relationship to the treatment of this condition.

Potentially Serious Consequences

With patience and persistence, spastic constipation can be managed successfully—and it's important to do so. If the condition remains untreated, it can progress to spastic colon, mucus colitis, spastic colitis, and even ulcerative colitis. For this reason, it is wise to take notice if your stools show evidence of mucus or traces of blood. Either of these, along with symptoms such as cramping and nausea, as well as episodes of explosive diarrhea, suggest the condition has progressed and you should visit your healthcare practitioner to obtain an accurate diagnosis and begin necessary treatment.

18. Asthma and Respiratory Disorders

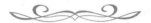

n the past three decades, the incidence of bronchial asthma has risen tenfold in the United States. Probably the most significant reason for this notable increase is exposure to larger amounts of environmental contaminants and pollutants. Indoor and outdoor allergens hamper the body's natural ability to prevent these toxic and irritating substances from being absorbed into the bloodstream, and for people whose immune systems are hypersensitive to environmental toxins, the result is congestion, inflammation, and swelling of the mucous membranes lining the nasal passageways, throat, bronchi and lungs. For some individuals, the result is acute and chronic bronchitis, recurring pneumonia, strep throat, tonsillitis, and even emphysema—in spite of sophisticated antibiotics and anti-inflammatories.

If you or someone you love has asthma, bronchitis, or any other recurrent lung disorder, the Golden Rules presented here will be very valuable.

CONVENTIONAL TREATMENTS

People with asthma typically use a variety of over-the-counter and prescription medications and inhalers to manage the condition. Some of these medications are more effective than others, but no matter how well they work, these products can only treat the symptoms—there is no cure. If non-steroidal medications offer little or no relief of asthma symptoms, doctors generally prescribe cortisone or prednisone, two very powerful steroid drugs that block the body's immune response. Because they are generally very effective in temporarily relieving the symptoms of asthma, many people become reliant on these steroid medications. Unfortunately, there can be serious consequences from their long-term use.

Side effects of extended steroid use include changes in body chemistry that can cause cataracts of the eyes, diabetes, facial bloating, fluid retention, high blood pressure, increased risk of infection, and osteoporosis. In addition, the adrenal glands—the source of natural cortisone in the body—stop producing this important hormone. Therefore, if you do use steroidal medications, be very careful about how you take them and how often you do so. Most alternative practitioners advise using such cortisone, prednisone, and related drugs only as a last resort.

ALTERNATIVE TREATMENT APPROACHES

Alternative strategies for managing asthma are available, and some are really quite simple. For example, a common source of irritation for people with asthma and chronic upper respiratory disorders is house dust from mites that live in dust and the fecal matter they produce. Although mites can live almost anywhere there is dust, they thrive in carpeting, draperies, furniture upholstery, mattresses, and pillows. Therefore, it may be helpful to buy covers for your mattress and pillows that are permeable to air and perspiration but impermeable to mites, and to wash your bed linen, curtains, and pajamas weekly in water that is hot enough to kill the mites. Also, because basements are often damp and are therefore prime areas for mold and fungus growth, people who have asthma should not sleep in a basement bedroom.

If your condition is particularly severe, the following suggestions may help you better manage your asthma or other respiratory condition:

- Avoid smoking and secondhand smoke entirely.

- Adapt and practice the breathing techniques described in Chapter 8.

- Do not use aspirin, ibuprofen, and other over-the-counter pain medications that can trigger severe asthma attacks. Acetaminophen products such as Tylenol are equally effective but safer to use for people with asthma.

- During the cold winter months, protect your nose and mouth with a scarf or cold-weather mask so that you do not breathe in very cold air, which can aggravate symptoms of respiratory disorders.

- Do not choose occupations that expose you to respiratory irritants and airborne contaminants.

- Consider purchasing an efficient air-filtration system. (See Chapter 8.)

- Control cockroaches by removing their food supply, which is usually food or garbage left out or in open containers. (The dust from their feces is a factor, as well as the remnant particles of their carcasses when they die.)

- Do not allow your pets to enter your bedroom.

- Do what you can to prevent colds and upper respiratory tract infections. (See Chapter 20 for more information on preventing these illnesses.)

- If you have a forced air furnace, change the filters regularly.

- Remove your bedroom carpeting and replace it with hardwood flooring.

- Use a humidifier that also provides air filtration in winter months.

- Use vacuum cleaners that trap dust and mites in a liquid medium.

Learn and Practice Stress Management

Reducing stress in your life can also help reduce symptoms of asthma and other respiratory conditions. Keep in mind that sources of stress may be chemical, emotional, physical, or spiritual, and each needs to be addressed equally. For most people, a combination of stressors cause illness. Your natural healthcare practitioner can work with you to help improve the function of your nervous system and immune system in responding to environmental and other stressors. Additionally, you may wish to work with a trained counselor to learn effective stress-management techniques and strategies.

Many chiropractors have reported dramatic alleviation of asthma—particularly in children and young adults—before its effects become chronic. Other non-drug-related health-enhancing considerations, such as aromatherapy, can also strengthen the overall function of your immune system and, therefore, your body as a whole.

Electro-Acupuncture by Voll—Electro-Dermal Screening

In Chapter 9, you learned about a system of body analysis known as electro-acupuncture by Voll, or electro-dermal screening (EDS). This amazing technology is particularly useful in accurately assessing and identifying environmental stressors related to a host of upper respiratory conditions, including allergies, bronchial asthma, sinusitis, and recurring infections. In many instances, the exact items to which the body is reacting negatively are identified and then eliminated through the use of homeopathic remedies. Many practitioners who use EDS and related treatment techniques have described exceptional results achieved by this subtle energy medicine.

19. Depression

~~~~~~~~~~~~~~~

most people can identify situations and events that trigger their states of sadness. And, as the situation responsible for those feelings passes with time, most people overcome their melancholy and are able to move on with their lives. This is known as situational depression. For others, however, when the events or situations that trigger bouts of sadness are overwhelming or unrelenting, the body, mind, and spirit are incapable of adjusting to the emotional demands placed upon them, and clinical depression is the result. This type of depression usually results from disturbances in the brain and endocrine system, which regulate our moods. Many factors can affect this disturbance. The Golden Rules and themes discussed in this chapter can help you alleviate the harsher edges of depression.

CLINICAL DEPRESSION— ILLNESS OF THE BODY, MIND, AND SPIRIT

Some of the world's most acclaimed and talented people struggle with clinical depression. It affects people of all ages, ethnicities, and genders from every walk of life, making most of us vulnerable. Approximately 25 percent of Americans suffer varying degrees of clinical depression at some point during their lives. Almost all depression results from a combination of factors, including drug or alcohol abuse, environmental factors, heredity, nutritional and hormonal imbalances, personal loss, side effects of medications, stress, and trauma—emotional, spiritual, or physical. In addition, depression often accompanies chronic illnesses, such as arthritis, cancer, diabetes, or debilitating heart or lung disease. For people who are depressed, the condition usually represents a significant amount of unhappiness and, in the most severe cases, results in bouts of total despair and disability, and may even end in suicide. Therefore, depression is not a casual concern, and you should be aware of the signs and symptoms so you will know if you or someone you love needs professional assistance. The following are the most common and well-known symptoms of major depression:

- Difficulty concentrating, remembering, or making decisions
- Disturbances in eating or sleeping patterns
- Extreme exhaustion and fatigue to the point of having no interest in ordinary activities, including social and sexual activity
- Feelings of guilt, helplessness, hopelessness, pessimism, or worthlessness
- Feeling persistently sad or empty
- Irritability, increased crying, anxiety, and panic attacks
- Loss of appetite
- Persistent physical symptoms, or aches and pains that do not respond to any treatment
- Abuse of alcohol, caffeine, drugs, food, nicotine, or other substances
- Thoughts of suicide, or suicide plans or attempts

Obviously, not everyone who is depressed will exhibit all of these symptoms, nor will they necessarily be the same in everyone. However, individuals who experience four or more of the above symptoms for more than two weeks are advised to seek professional attention. If you are often struck by sadness and find yourself feeling trapped in a very difficult emotional space, it's important to take these concerns to a professional.

It is becoming increasingly clear that depression can result from biochemical imbalances that affect the way the brain works. Today, about 80 percent of depression can be effectively managed with special medications and carefully chosen nutrients that can help balance the brain's chemistry. For example, studies have shown that 80 percent of those living with clinical depression had an underlying magnesium deficiency. Allergies, environmental toxicity, and food sensitivities can also play a major role in brain chemistry, and should be taken into consideration in any diagnosis of depression. Finally, professional counseling is a very important component of treatment and recovery. By focusing on the need for harmony within the body, mind, and spirit, a holistically oriented practitioner can help you to understand and eventually overcome many of your concerns.

Alternative Considerations

In addition to seeking conventional Western medical intervention, people who are predisposed to depression should pay particular attention to the factors mentioned above that can affect their brain chemistry. Be mindful of the purity of the air you breathe, the water you drink, and the foods you eat, and pay special attention to the thoughts you think.

Your brain can be no healthier than the rest of your body. If you neglect your physical health, you may also be neglecting your brain function. For example, the world-renowned painter Vincent Van Gogh, who committed suicide at a young age, had a blinding eye disease known as glaucoma, and many believe that toward the end of his life he gradually went insane. One of his habits was to keep the tips of his paintbrushes sharp by repeatedly placing them in his mouth every few brush strokes. It is now known that the pigment in red paint contains cadmium, which is highly toxic to the brain and nervous system. In addition, many of the paints used in earlier times contained lead, another potent poison and neurotoxin. These factors, alone or in combination, could well have been responsible for his final mental state. Ludwig van Beethoven, the world-famous composer, also died of lead poisoning. In addition to gradually becoming totally deaf, it is said he suffered severe mood swings and depression, and exhibited serious anti-social behavior prior to his death. Recent evaluation of preserved locks of his hair demonstrated seven times the normal limits of lead in his chemistry.

A growing list of safe, naturally occurring herbal remedies have been proven helpful in managing clinical depression. In addition to aiding in the treatment of arthritis, as mentioned earlier, SAM-e (S-adenosylmethionine) can be effective in treating some forms of depression. Likewise, St. John's wort is an herb that has been shown to help safely and naturally alleviate depression; in fact, doctors in Germany prescribe St. John's wort twenty-five times more than Prozac. A word of caution is in order, however, for those who choose to try natural agents to treat depression. Some herbal and other natural products may actually have harmful interactions with prescription medications. For example, St. John's wort should not be taken in combination with certain mood-altering prescription medications such as Prozac and Zoloft.

Work Can Be Therapeutic

Perhaps you have heard of the emotional struggles that President Abraham Lincoln faced during the Civil War. Having battled the demons of depression for most of his life, President Lincoln fell into periods of despair during the darkest days of the war when he felt totally incapacitated and incapable of providing the kind of leadership that the country so desperately needed. In his memoirs, Lincoln reflected upon how he would struggle through these difficult times by pick-ing up an axe and splitting wood. He wrote that there was nothing more pow-erful or effective to help him break the cycle of disabling depression than three or four hours of vigorous manual labor, sometimes over several days in a row.

Those around Mr. Lincoln believed he was out splitting wood simply to divert his mind from his worries; indeed, part of the benefit of this type of activ-ity may have been the mental diversion that physical labor offered. Since 1973, scientists have known that physically activating the body through work or vig-orous exercise stimulates the production of endorphins, naturally occurring opiates secreted by the brain that reduce the experience of pain. In addition, as scientists discovered later, the body also secretes related molecules called en-kephalins as the result of physical exertion. Enkephalins have the effect of ele-vating mood, thereby helping to alleviate feelings of depression.

SEASONAL AFFECTIVE DISORDER (SAD)

A less understood condition that causes depression is seasonal affective disorder (SAD), brought about by lack of adequate sunlight. SAD is also referred to as "winter depression" because it develops in the darker winter months, particu-larly in parts of the world with a colder climate, and it lasts for the duration of the winter season. Symptoms of the condition include anxiety, irritability, loss of interest in activities, moodiness, weight gain, cravings for sweets and alcohol, crying spells, fatigue, headaches, and insomnia. Studies indicate that as many as 5 percent of Americans have this disorder, with people between eighteen and thirty years of age at greatest risk of developing the condition.

Treatment for SAD is light therapy—sunlight if it's available, artificial light provided by ultraviolet bulbs if natural light is not adequate. If you feel that your life is affected by SAD, make an effort to get more sunshine or exposure to ultra-violet light in the darker days of winter. Exercise, stress management, and nutri-tional supplements that stimulate the production of the brain chemical serotonin are also beneficial in treating SAD.

SPECIAL CONCERN FOR TEENAGE DEPRESSION

While older people are at significant risk for depression, one of the most tragic events we can experience is the untimely death of a young person, and when the death is self-inflicted, the tragedy is compounded. Depression is the cause of more than two-thirds of the 30,000 reported suicides in the United States each year, and of these, about eight to eleven out of every 100,000 are teenagers—a figure equal to that for teenagers who die from all other natural causes combined.

Depression is the most common emotional problem experienced during adolescence and it is the single greatest risk factor for suicide among adolescents. The National Institute of Mental Health estimates that up to 8 percent of American teenagers experience major depression, and girls are twice as vulnerable as boys. According to a 1999 survey, about 20 percent of high school students have seriously considered suicide.

Most often, depression is a treatable biological disease resulting from an imbalance of brain chemicals. The warning signs of teen depression are similar to those described above for adults. Unfortunately, peer pressure during teenage years tends to magnify the perception of sadness and despair with which many young people struggle and they may not understand or believe that things can get better as they age.

What Parents Need to Do

If you are the parent of a teenager who exhibits the warning signs of depression described at the beginning of this chapter, it's important to take your child to a professional who can promptly and accurately diagnose the condition. Remember, it's imperative to take this matter very seriously—your actions may very well save your child's life. The following recommendations can guide you in helping your child to recover from depression:

- Keep channels of communication open. Let your child know that your love is unconditional and you will always be there.

- Don't assume that bouts of moodiness and sadness always represent a normal "phase" all youngsters go through.

- Seek professional help early—the sooner the condition is accurately diagnosed and appropriately treated, the better.

- Carefully inventory and remove all potentially dangerous medications from convenient locations in your household.

- Remove all guns and other weapons from the home that could be used impulsively in acts of self-destruction.

- Have the courage to confront your child about the possible use or abuse of drugs and alcohol. Alcohol is a serious depressant that's readily accessible to most teenagers, and it has a cumulative negative effect on brain function. Illegal substances such as marijuana, while initially tranquilizing, can also have a depressive effect.

- Consider the possibility that your child could benefit from a broad holistic approach that could include special attention to diet and lifestyle issues.

Additionally, it's important to remember that a variety of physical disorders can cause or complicate emotional disorders. For example, take a moment to review the symptoms of low-blood sugar, or hypoglycemia, presented in Chapter 12. Also, a deficiency of the mineral magnesium, as well as inadequate consumption of essential oils and fatty acids, has been strongly linked to depression and other mental health disorders. To learn more about the role of essential oils in mental health disorders, I recommend you read the extraordinary book *Smart Fats* by Dr. Michael Schmidt.

Finally, in my professional experience, I have found that clinical depression, as well as other mental health conditions in adults or teenagers, may be helped by the Electro-Dermal Screening (EDS), initially described in Chapter 9. This simple, inexpensive, and sophisticated system of testing can determine damaging agents in the environment or accumulated in the brain and nervous system that can be eliminated with safe, effective homeopathic remedies, and followed up with specific nutritional support.

Disabling depression has the potential to become suicidal despair. The opposite of despair is hope. You can help your child recover a feeling of hope. In doing so, you may wish to emphasize spiritual considerations and a belief and faith in a higher power that becomes a source of loving acceptance and hope. This is true for adult depression as well.

Additional Resources

A new questionnaire test, available nationwide through the Youth Depression Screening Initiative, allows kids to hear questions over headphones and respond in complete privacy via computers. The Center for the Advancement of Children's Mental Health at Columbia University is working with schools and communities to administer the test and provide follow-up treatment, if indicated. For more information about this service, visit their website at www.kidsmentalhealth.org. In addition, the National Mental Health Awareness Campaign provides resources to help people overcome various mental illnesses at www.nostigma.org.

For teens and adults troubled by depression and suicidal thoughts, a national patient advocacy group called the Depression and Bipolar Support Alliance is distributing a free, wallet-sized card that lists a suicide prevention hotline number: 1-800-442-4673. The card is available by calling 1-800-826-3632, or visit the Alliance's website at www.dbsalliance.org.

20. Colds, Flu, and Other Infections

Common colds and influenza result in more workplace absences than any other illness. Every year, Americans lose millions of work days, experience significant distress and misery, and spend billions of dollars on cold and flu remedies.

UNDERSTANDING COLDS AND FLU

With all the advances made in medical science, and all of modern medicine's wonder drugs and high-tech interventions, it seems as if we have yet to identify effective ways to treat the common cold or simple influenza. One of my well-known and highly respected colleagues recently stated his conviction that there will never be a cure for the common cold. He even speculates that the cold *is* the cure, meaning that cold and flu symptoms may actually be the body's means of detoxification. In other words, the coughing, fever, sneezing, and sniffling of the common cold, and the aches, pains, diarrhea, and vomiting that accompany influenza are the body's efforts at purging itself. My colleague's belief is that the cold results from the body wisely choosing to stay in balance with its environment—an interesting theory that is aligned with traditional Chinese medicine (TCM). You can certainly appreciate that colds, flu, and related fatigue do force us to slow down and rest, allowing time to take stock as to why and how the immune system has failed to resist these common viruses. Taking this more holistic approach to finding solutions for colds and flu reminds us of how the body is attuned to self-regulate and remain in harmony for the ultimate purpose of survival.

Antibiotics and Cold and Flu Viruses

Colds and flu are the result of opportunistic viruses that have overcome the body's resistance when the immune system is not functioning at its peak. Antibiotics have absolutely no killing effect on viral infections and do not, therefore, have a place in the prevention and treatment of colds and flu.

Prevention Is the Key

If you suffer from recurring colds, flu, and other respiratory infections, you would do well to review the many suggestions presented throughout this book that can help you maintain and enhance immune system function. You will recall the importance of keeping your body chemistry alkaline, and the great value of powerful germ-fighting foods such as garlic, onion, cider vinegar, raw honey, bee pollen, and royal jelly. Vitamins A and C, as well as the mineral zinc, are key in maintaining the health and integrity of the mucous membranes of the body, while the mineral colloidal silver—taken only in small doses for a short time— is a powerful germ fighter that destroys viruses and other harmful organisms. Echinacea and goldenseal are two important herbs that also aid in the treatment and prevention of the common cold. And, yes, your grandmother was correct in telling you that chicken soup has ingredients that can help cure the common cold.

To overcome colds and flu, it's important to stay warm enough to induce perspiration, obtain adequate sleep and rest, avoid alcohol and nicotine, and minimize caffeine intake. You should also drink plenty of pure water; consume fresh fruits, vegetables, and their juices; avoid excessive physical, emotional, and spiritual stress; and practice the Golden Rules outlined in this book. Additionally, many of the recommended treatments for colds and flu listed above can actually help prevent these illnesses.

GERMS—FRIEND OR FOE?

It is important to remember that germs, those microscopic little creatures sharing the earth with us, are critically important in maintaining and preserving our life on the planet. Of course bacteria, fungi, parasites, rickettsia, viruses, and other germs can play a role in various human and animal diseases, but I wish to emphasize that the primary role of microorganisms on the earth is to participate in the breakdown of dying, decaying, and dead organic matter into its original elements so that it can be "recycled."

As you know, everything alive will eventually die—every animal on land or sea, every blade of grass and every tree, and every human being. Can you imagine the earth if the carcass of every living species ever born were to remain here after it died? If this happened, there would be no room for anything but the unchanging remains of these dead creatures. Can you now better appreciate the role of microorganisms? If you walk through a forest, you will see dozens of trees and large branches that have fallen to the earth and are in various stages of decay, evidence of millions of microbes doing their job. When the microbes have completed their task, the resulting organic mulch becomes a rich humus base for future vegetative growth, including new trees from which the mulch came—an excellent example of nature's energies being recycled.

The same is true regarding our own existence. Pioneering research in this field is expressed in *Blueprint for Immortality,* the fascinating work of Dr. Harold Saxon Burr, who demonstrated that all life is essentially electrical in nature. His research expresses some of the early, practical applications of the quantum physics/mechanics theories and principles explored by Niels Bohr, Albert Einstein, Werner Heisenberg, Erwin Schrodinger, and others. With very sensitive electrical-detection instruments, Dr. Burr was able to predict which trees in a forest were dying, as many as three years before they showed any external signs of this happening. This was possible because healthy trees emanate a healthy frequency, but as a tree begins to die, the wavelengths and energy field surrounding it begin to change. More recent, highly provocative research takes this information to the next level, showing how the same is true for humans. Dr. Robert Becker, a world-famous orthopedic surgeon and researcher, has shown that electrical frequencies relate directly to the repair of bone fractures and to cell regeneration. Anyone interested in further exploring this subject should read Dr. Becker's work *The Body Electric.* Other books, such as *Vibrational Medicine* and *A Practical Guide to Vibrational Medicine* by Richard Gerber, M.D., and *Quantum Healing* by Deepak Chopra, M.D., provide additional, exciting information regarding this area of science. If you want to learn more about quantum physics and how understanding and applying these new sciences not only affects our health and well-being, but virtually every aspect of our lives, you will enjoy *The Field* by Lynne McTaggart. This book, the product of eight years of careful research, represents an enlightening journey into the world of quantum mechanics and the future of science.

These areas of scientific discovery are based upon the theory that microorganisms can detect the resonant frequencies of healthy tissues, as well as the dissonant frequencies of unhealthy body tissues. It's believed that microbes are drawn to only unhealthy tissues, those with out-of-balance, discordant electrical energies, representing the first stages of the death for these cells. In keeping with nature's purpose, microbes are attracted to the area to begin the cleanup process and assure further tissue decomposition. Given this thesis, we can begin to understand that germs are not necessarily harmful, or a threat to life on earth.

Further, as you can now better appreciate, the real secret to avoiding the potentially harmful consequences of germs in and on your body is to keep your tissue cells maximally healthy and emanating only positive, healthy frequencies.

The Body Electric—Healthy Vibes

Many different factors influence the human body's resonant frequencies, including our diet, air and water quality, clothing, housing, and sewage disposal. In addition, lifestyle factors, such as the use of toxic substances like alcohol, nicotine, and other drugs, and even the thoughts that we think and the beliefs and attitudes we hold, seem to affect our vibes. This helps to explain why, in a classroom of thirty students, there will be several children who are repeatedly ill and others who are almost never sick. Although all of the students are exposed to the same harmful, contagious germs, some seem much more vulnerable to illness, while others are almost never ill.

Understanding the body as essentially an electrical phenomenon also explains why certain people seem to give off positive energy. These are people that others are likely attracted to because they find a balancing, calming, and healing quality in their presence. Along these lines, people whose vibrations are discordant or negative may actually have a repulsive quality, causing others to shun them. Not surprisingly, as a result of this isolation, a person who gives off negative energy is also more vulnerable to depression and disharmony in body, mind, and spirit—a set of circumstances that eventually sets the stage for the development of a wide variety of illnesses and disease. For further insight into this topic, I urge you to read *Molecules of Emotion* by Candace Pert, Ph.D.

Let Your Children Play in the Dirt

People who are overly conscientious about avoiding common household and playground germs are often *more* likely to develop infections. This is because, through repeated exposures to germs of all types in small doses, a healthy immune system is stimulated to produce naturally occurring antibodies. Constantly using antibacterial soaps, antiseptic sprays, cleaners, and mouthwashes may actually contribute to lowering your resistance to colds, flu, and other infectious illnesses. So, all you parents out there, take note: it's okay to let your children play in the mud and get themselves dirty. You can relax and trust the body's natural inborn wisdom to protect itself. This is not to suggest that you should neglect your children's personal hygiene and, obviously, unnecessary or intentional exposure to serious contagious diseases is not appropriate for anyone of any age group. Let common sense guide you.

Keeping your immune system strong and healthy is certainly your best defense against germ-causing diseases. On his deathbed, Louis Pasteur, one of the greatest microbiologists of all time, is said to have conceded to his colleagues that the emphasis should not be on the germ, but rather on the "soil of the host." Pasteur recognized that, as long as the cells of the host organism—plant, animal, or human—are strong and resilient and the immune system is healthy, the "harmful" organism would usually do no harm. The Golden Rules presented in this book will help you keep your immune system in top shape to protect your body against illness.

BACTERIAL INFECTIONS— ANTIBIOTICS AND GERMS

Antibiotics are truly an example of miracle medicines saving millions and millions of lives. Because this is true, however, there has been a tendency in Western cultures to overuse antibiotics and even use them inappropriately, to the point that public health authorities have grave concerns about the growing number of antibiotic-resistant strains of deadly mutant organisms that are developing. Although antibiotics can kill a wide variety of potentially life-threatening germs, they do so indiscriminately, while also destroying the normal, beneficial bacterial flora in the intestinal tract. In addition, since antibiotics have absolutely no killing effect on fungi, viruses, or yeast, they can indirectly allow for the increased possibility of infection from one of these microbes. In light of all these risks, it is recommended that you use antibiotics only when absolutely necessary.

Candidiasis is an excellent example of a common yeast infection resulting from overuse of antibiotics. The infection commonly manifests as athlete's foot; fingernail or toenail fungus; thrush of the gums, mouth, or tongue; jock itch; or vaginitis. For people whose immune systems are impaired, candidiasis can also cause a stubborn systemic infection that affects all the organs and systems of the body. A diet high in refined sugar and yeast products also increases the likelihood of candidiasis infection.

Probiotics

Probiotics are naturally occurring agents that help restore normal, healthy flora in the gut. If you do need to take antibiotics, be sure to take the medications as directed, and then follow up with cultured yogurt, lactobacillus, acidophilus, or bifidus tablets to restore the natural intestinal bacterial flora. You should also avoid refined sugar and products containing yeast during treatment with antibiotics to minimize the risk of candidiasis and other yeast infections.

As an alternative to antibiotics, there are many safe, effective homeopathic remedies for combating harmful microbes.

ADDITIONAL RESOURCES

For a more comprehensive review of natural approaches to the clinical management and prevention of microbial infections, you will enjoy reading *Beyond Antibiotics* by Dr. Michael Schmidt. If you are interested in exploring more material on electromagnetic energy fields and health, I encourage you to read *Electrical Nutrition* by Denie and Shelley Hiestand. This enlightening book also discusses the integrity of the immune system and the prevention of disease through natural means.

In summary, while research has not yet hit upon a cure for the common cold and other resistant organisms, a growing body of evidence suggests that colds, flu, and the majority of bacterial infections can be prevented. Much can also be done to reduce the frequency and severity of colds, flu, and other infections if all attempts at prevention fail. It's as simple as following the Golden Rules.

21. Stress Management

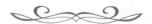

nderstanding stress is the first step in improving your ability to cope during times of adversity and challenge in your life. Consider the following definition from *Blakiston's New Gould Medical Dictionary, 2nd Edition:*

> [Stress is] any stimulus or succession of stimuli of such magnitude as to tend to disrupt the homeostasis (harmony) of the organism; when mechanisms of adjustment fail or become disproportionate or incoordinate, the stress may be considered an injury, resulting in disease, disability, and death.

From this, it's clear how unrelenting stress can directly or indirectly cause illness and may eventually result in death. Even if stress has not yet resulted in full-blown disease, for many people, it has significantly contributed to misery in their lives.

STRESS CAN BE A LIFESAVER

It's important to keep in mind that short episodes of stress and anxiety are normal and can be critically important to your health and survival. If you have just dealt with an extremely stressful event, such as a life-threatening experience, it's natural to notice physical symptoms such as clammy hands, diarrhea, lightheadedness, a lump in your throat, nausea or queasiness, rapid pulse rate, shaking, sweating, and trembling. These are your body's innate protective mechanisms that prevent you from repeating the same mistakes or intentionally encountering the same dangers, and such physical responses usually disappear once the source of the real (or perceived) danger has passed. It's nature's way of reminding us to pay more attention to what's going on around us, change the way we make decisions or change the decisions we make, shift our attitudes, and learn ways of coping during times of adversity. Seeking instant relief from

drinking alcohol; binge eating; taking mood elevators, sleeping pills, or tranquilizers; and engaging in other risky behaviors will only add stress to your life
in the long run.

Interestingly, perceived dangers elicit the same physical responses as genuine threats to our existence. Therefore, it's important to carefully assess the
validity of the circumstances you believe to be threatening, because what you
perceive to be real could become your reality and, even when founded upon
false beliefs, may cause grave harm.

THE LINK BETWEEN DIET AND STRESS

You may have noticed that the word "desserts" spelled backwards is "stressed."
Is there a relationship between what you eat and feelings of stress? Yes, indeed.
There is a great deal of evidence to show that overloading the body with sugar
and other refined starches found in desserts such as candy, cookies, pastries, and
so forth can disturb the body's glucose balance and cause hypoglycemia (low
blood sugar), a condition we initially discussed in Chapter 12. Drinking alcohol
and soda has the same effect. You may recall that the symptoms of hypoglycemia include anxiety, depression, dizziness, emotional upset, exhaustion, a
feeling of faintness or blackout sensation, fatigue, headaches, inability to concentrate, insomnia, irritability, mood swings, nervousness, shakiness, and weakness when hungry—all symptoms that may seem similar to those you experience
when you're under pressure. Therefore, you may want to carefully reconsider
your intake of desserts and other sugary or starchy foods if you wish to more
effectively manage any stress in your life.

OVERCOMING STRESS

In addition to the many suggestions offered throughout this book for managing
stress and maintaining good health in general—getting enough sleep, exercising,
taking walks, meditating, eating a healthy diet, and practicing yoga, to name a
few—the following recommendations can also help you combat stress and
improve the quality of your life.

Learn to Welcome Change

Think about this: You do not have to improve to change, but you do have to
change to improve. An unwillingness or inability to adapt to changes in your life
can cause you to experience a great deal of unnecessary stress, mainly because
you may feel that you are not in control of the situation. Learn to welcome

changes in your life—change prevents our lives from quickly becoming boring, dull, and stagnant.

Find a Hobby

As with any activity that diverts your attention from the many stresses of day-to-day life, enjoyable hobbies can be a soul-satisfying diversion from the daily grind and, therefore, an excellent means of stress reduction. The list of hobbies is as long as your imagination: antiquing, athletics, boating, camping, collecting coins or stamps, fishing, gardening, hiking, playing or enjoying music, painting and drawing, studying photography, and exploring acting or visiting the theater can benefit you emotionally, physically, and spiritually. In addition to being a pleasant diversion from stress, volunteer work can also be highly rewarding because you are helping others in addition to helping yourself, so you may wish to participate in community service, church, or civic activities in your area, or find ways to assist young people in need of a mentor or older individuals who are longing for company and care. Finally, taking care of one or more pets can also be an enjoyable and rewarding experience that will keep you from focusing on more negative aspects of your life.

Give Up the Need to Resist

In the Eastern traditions, it is believed that stress results only from resisting what is happening in our lives. With this in mind, try to remember that the circumstances of your life and the lives of your loved ones are occurring just as they should and happening precisely on schedule. Reflect on the possibility that everything you experience is happening for your spiritual advancement, as tests of our love and strength. Doubt arises because we don't know the whole story, but keep in mind that life is like a tapestry and, as we should not focus on the individual threads in the fabric, we should not focus on the minor events of our lives, but must instead trust that the big picture—the tapestry—appears as it should. Many times, what appears to be bad news turns out to be for the best in the long run. Therefore, in matters that you do not readily understand, it's important to stay flexible, go with the flow, and then exercise trust in a higher power to guide you, and have great faith in the outcome.

Make Good Use of Your Time

Learning how to reasonably manage your time can greatly reduce the stress you experience in your daily living. As you plan your day, try to leave room for interruptions and distractions, because doing so allows chance to act positively in your life. After all, there is no accurate way to predict when the next great opportunity may come knocking on your door. Remember Emily Dickinson's adage, "The soul should always stand ajar, ready to welcome the ecstatic experience."

Further Your Education

Education is the single most important key to prosperity, understanding and, many times, good health. In Western societies, formal education is readily available and mostly affordable. While it's true that education can be expensive, by contrast, consider the price of ignorance. If you lack the time or funds to advance your education in the classroom, remember that self-education and self-awareness can also be invaluable in your life journey—and it's as accessible and inexpensive as your local public library. Actively seek out reliable self-help health information. Selectively use your television time for educational purposes. Take advantage of the many educational resources available on the Internet. Take time to read because, after all, the person who does not read is no better off than the person who cannot read. In all your activities, listen, learn, and apply what you need.

Express Your Sadness

All of us feel sad from time to time, and it's healthy to express those feelings. Following any major loss or trauma in your life, it's important to grieve and, in fact, crying can be a highly effective stress-reliever. Author and philosopher Natalie Barney said, "Time engraves our faces with all the tears we have not shed." It's also okay—indeed, it's important—to accept the inevitable. Looking to a power greater than yourself can help you find profound peace and can become an important first step in your ability to carry on with the rest of your life.

Live to Laugh

There is probably no more effective stress relief than laughter. Funny movies and videos, stand-up comedy, and humorous books, articles, and television programs produce deep, hearty laughter than can help relieve stress and, as a result, improve the functioning of your immune and endocrine systems. Clearly, then, laughter is of enormous value for your whole being—body, mind, and spirit. So as often as possible, try to have a belly-rocking, thigh-slapping, tears-rolling laugh.

Did you know that, on average, kids laugh up to 400 times each day, while the average adult laughs only 15 times a day? Cherish your inner child. Nurture your natural, inborn sense of humor by learning to take life less seriously, and don't forget to laugh at yourself from time to time. If you would like to have more

Laughing Matters

A middle-aged man was concerned that his wife might be losing her hearing and paid a visit to his doctor. The doctor, explaining that this could indeed be a very serious handicap, said it was proper to be concerned. He told the man what to do to test his suspicions. So, that evening when the man returned home from work, he entered the front door, saw his wife at the kitchen stove preparing food and, just as the doctor suggested, he approached quietly. At about ten feet from his wife, he asked in a louder-than-usual voice, "Honey, what's for dinner?" Silence. Not a sound. No response at all. Even more concerned by this time, he walked to within five feet of his wife and, in an even louder voice, repeated, "Honey, what's for dinner?" Once again, no response. By now extremely concerned, he came right up behind her and shouted in her ear, "Honey, what's for dinner?" She turned, fixed him with a look, and said, "For the third time, I said meat loaf, you deaf donkey!"

friends and be welcomed in almost any crowd, become a source of tasteful humor. Like any other art form, learning how to tell funny stories and harmless jokes takes practice and timing, but the rewards can last a lifetime. Laughter can greatly expand your enjoyment and extend your life *and* the lives of others.

Work and Stress vs. Work and Stress Relief

There is an axiom in occupational health circles that says, "Work is therapeutic." If you are one of the many people who does not enjoy your job, perhaps you would not agree. For your own happiness and success, however, it's very important to love what you do for a living. My friend Joe Batten coined the phrase for the U.S. Army, "Be all that you can be." But if you don't love your work, how can you be at your very best? Everyone deserves the rewards of meaningful work that bestows a great sense of personal joy and satisfaction. Your work, and every task you accomplish, reflects you and your inner character. And it's amazing how much can get done, and how much progress you can make, when it doesn't matter who gets the credit. In his classic work *The Prophet*, the Lebanese philosopher Kahlil Gibran says, "Work is love made visible." Whatever you do for a living, give it your all; but if you are truly unhappy in your career, it might be better—for your mental and, ultimately, physical health—to pursue a different path. And remember, if you wish to earn the good will and gratitude of those with whom you work, it's better to under-promise and over-deliver than to over-promise and under-deliver.

If you have the physical energy and emotional capacity to do so, you may find that your health in body, mind, and spirit would benefit from doing additional service. Obviously, if you are a working mother with three small children, spending forty or more hours each week away from your family would not be the best way to live a balanced life. Each individual needs to carefully consider the amount of time he or she can realistically devote to work activities that provide income and security for themselves and their family members.

If you work nights or the late shift, you should be aware that working these hours can be a major source of illness, injury, and stress. Throughout many centuries of evolvement, our sleep and waking patterns have adapted to the circadian rhythm, the cycles of sunlight during the day and darkness during the night. If your occupation requires you to remain awake and work through the night, you may be surprised to learn that your health may suffer as your body tries to readjust to an unnatural circadian rhythm. While some individuals are "night people" who may actually prefer working irregular hours, when they feel more energetic, comfortable, and efficient, this seems to be the exception, not the rule. Most studies have shown that night-shift workers suffer more illnesses and experience more stress than traditional day workers, with symptoms such as digestive disturbances, headaches, heart and circulatory problems, insomnia, nervous system disorders, or social problems.

Employers need to be concerned about the health consequences of working at night, and provide employees with more choice regarding the shifts they are expected to work. If you are a shift worker who is sensitive to circadian rhythm disturbances, you should speak with your employer so that the most suitable arrangement can be found. Additionally, you may be surprised to learn that working night-shift schedules for months, or even years, is actually less stressful than adapting to new work shifts every few weeks. Therefore, employers must be careful not to schedule their employees for short periods of night-shift work followed by short periods of daytime work.

If you are feeling the ill health effects of shift work, it's important to raise this issue with your employer. If your employer does not want to make any changes in your work schedule, you may need to consider changing jobs, or perhaps asking your doctor to intervene with your employer on your behalf. Your employer is obligated to make reasonable accommodations for your needs if your doctor finds that your work schedule is negatively impacting your health.

Remember to Play

As essential as soul-satisfying work is in managing stress, it's equally important to leave room for playtime in your life. The beckoning spirit of childhood is too often ignored in our demanding society. Rediscover the tingle of the crack of the bat, the bang of the firecracker, the delightful splash created as you dove into your favorite swimming hole as a child. If it's been some time since you've felt the wind in your hair from the old tire swing, or the thrill of sliding into home plate, it's probably time to become reacquainted with your inner child.

Even as an adult, you will find that there are many "playtime" activities to embrace as your spirit moves you. Go antique shopping, bowling, fishing, or dancing; play tennis, golf, or billiards; lace up your roller skates and hit the roller rink or slip into your bathing suit and dive into the pool. Use your imagination. Your inner child will thank you with better sleep, a healthy appetite for tomorrow, a stronger immune system, and a renewed zest for living. And remember this: we don't stop playing because we grow old, we grow old because we stop playing.

Learn to Take Risks

Henry David Thoreau once wrote, "Most men lead lives of quiet desperation and go to the grave with the song still in them." More simply put, "He who hesitates is lost." While it's certainly wise to live prudently and responsibly, it's also important to take some risks from time to time. The greater the risk, the greater the reward—and your life may be the better for it.

Become a Student of Human Nature

Mark Twain said, "There's a lot of human nature in people." With this in mind, realize that everyone you encounter in your life is a teacher in your lifelong study of human nature, and every encounter is a lesson. When other people's attitudes, behavior, or beliefs seem incomprehensible, remind yourself that the actions and words of others don't have to make sense to you. Many times, they don't even make sense to the people themselves.

Everyone and everything is a direct reflection of how you see the world. As you are, you see others. As you see others, you are. When you step out of the role of judge and into the role of quiet observer, this rule will become quite clear to you. Remember the words of Will Rogers, who said, "I have never known anyone well enough to be able to judge him."

Practice Yoga

Yoga incorporates exercise and stretching, mental discipline, proper breathing, and techniques to improve posture, and it's an excellent and enjoyable way to reduce stress and improve your physical and spiritual health. Because yoga offers so many health benefits, it's small wonder that it has become so popular in recent years, with more and more yoga studios opening all the time. If you decide that you would like to try yoga as a means of improving your physical health and mental well-being, be sure to start out slowly and carefully. Some yoga postures are quite advanced, and can result in injury if you are not physically ready to tackle them.

Try Meditation

Practicing meditation allows you to spend time in that quiet place within, to seek out your still point—and its health and stress-reduction benefits are nothing short of incredible. What should you consciously experience when you are meditating? Absolutely nothing. That's the whole idea. Meditation allows you to access that special place between your thoughts, a place that is occupied by the infinite. By practicing meditation, you will be able to enter the realm of infinite possibilities.

Try an experiment: Stop thinking for the next sixty seconds. How did you do? Quite frustrating, isn't it? For most, it requires a supreme act of will to overcome the mind's ceaseless chatter. In fact, for most people, the harder they try, the more frustrating the effort becomes. By participating in this futile effort we learn what meditation is not. Meditation is *not* what you think.

Many different meditation techniques are practiced by millions of people every day, and they all, no doubt, have value. My personal favorite is transcendental meditation (TM), which requires formal training and, thus, a greater investment of time and resources to learn. However, there is an impressive amount of scientific evidence documenting the wide range of health benefits that TM offers.

Learn to Live in the Moment

It may surprise you to learn that the symptom patients most frequently describe to doctors is fatigue, and in most cases, there is no established disease condition to explain it. Many experts believe that the cause of fatigue is primarily psychological, and stress may be a factor. It seems that one of the explanations for why many people are chronically fatigued is that they try to live three days at a time. For some reason, people are inclined to relive and regret yesterday, and worry and fret about tomorrow, leaving very little energy to enjoy the wonders and beauty of today.

Learn to live in the present moment—it's all you have. Resolve to live joyfully, gratefully, and passionately each day. As Wendell Barry wrote in his poem *Mad Farmer,* "Be joyful, even though you know all the facts." Consider, too, that moments are different than minutes. Minutes have square edges and defined parameters, like being confined in a box. Moments have soft edges and are not defined or confining. Moments can be extended into infinity. They really have little to do with time, and much more to do with attitude.

Much unhappiness is caused by shifting your consciousness from the only reality that exists, which is *now,* to events from the past or fears of the future, neither of which has reality for the present. *The Power of Now* by Eckhart Tolle is an exceptional book that discusses the importance of remaining focused on the present moment. Tolle provides highly persuasive information on the joy and wonder of living in the present, and clearly states the danger of allowing your undisciplined thoughts to erode and damage your life in all its aspects—emotional, physical, and spiritual. In reflecting on the importance of living each day to its fullest, remember this quote: "The good news is that you don't need another thousand years to become free. All you need is to become present to this moment; to open yourself up to the fullness that already is, *now.*"

Don't become a casualty on the mind's babble field. The mind requires constant discipline. Disciplined minds can be the greatest instruments of creativity, inspiration, and joy on earth. Undisciplined minds can be the greatest source of sadness, tragedy, and violence on earth. The choice is yours.

Bring Harmony into Your Relationships

There are really only three relationships you must be concerned about—your relationships with yourself, your fellow humans, and your higher power. Of course, for all these, love is the key. Every creed, philosophy, religion, or other source of spiritual guidance agrees that the grand solution to all human problems is unconditional love. However, for many people, moving from an emotional state of bitterness and hatred, deep-seated anger, or resentment, to a sense of all-embracing love is not an easy task.

Often, when things don't go right in our lives, people tend to blame God or the powers that be. The "it's not fair" refrain is more popular than you might think among individuals who believe they were singled out to experience only sad events in this life. If you catch yourself dwelling on the "Why me?" mode of thought, ask yourself if this isn't just another convenient excuse for not wanting to take responsibility for your life.

Tolerance is a good place to start working toward the ultimate goal of being able to love unconditionally. From that point, you can proceed to the next stage, forgiveness, followed by respect, then admiration, friendship, trust, and perhaps, over a long period of time, the crown jewel itself—love. A simple yet powerful statement on which to reflect is, "I love you, not because you are good, but because I am good." Think about the deeper meaning of this: "I love you, not because you are good (or what you do or did is good), but because I realize that if I hate you, the hatred I feel will do me much more harm than it will you." To continue hating your enemies would clearly place your harmony of body, mind, and spirit in great peril. Therefore love is the means, as well as the end.

For sound health in mind, body, and spirit, it is important to develop tolerance toward your neighbor, and here the word "neighbor" refers not only to the people in your neighborhood, but to the entire human family. Tolerance can begin passively, with little or no true effort on your part, but to gain a true sense of peace within your soul, you must also actively practice tolerance. Go beyond the minimum of simply developing an understanding, and make a decision to share your understanding of attitudinal, cultural, and religious differences. Doing this can be wonderfully rewarding to the spirit, as you experience for yourself the peace that is possible when you step out of the role of judge.

Tolerance, forgiveness, and loving acceptance of self are, for many, even more difficult and challenging than learning to love others. You cannot give what you do not have. It is difficult to see any beauty and wisdom in other people if you cannot see these traits in yourself. Realistic love for yourself is neither vain nor arrogant; instead, it's an important way of honoring and showing gratitude for the precious gift of your unique, one-of-a-kind self. In all your thoughts and life activities, learn ways to improve for the sake of your health and happiness. And remember that, as with learning to love others, learning to love yourself takes tolerance and patience, as well. In *The Power of Now*, Eckhart Tolle writes, "Many people live with a tormentor in their head that continuously attacks and punishes them and drains them of their vital energy. It is the cause of untold misery and unhappiness." Don't let that happen to you.

THE HOLMES-RAHE STRESS INVENTORY

From time to time, it may be a good idea to identify and re-examine the sources of stress in your life. Back in the 1950s, Dr. Thomas Holmes, a psychiatrist at the University of Washington, devised the Holmes-Rahe Social Readjustment Rating Scale after observing that the single common denominator for the development of stress was "the necessity of significant change in the life pattern of an individual." He found that, among tuberculosis patients, the onset of the disease generally followed a series of challenging personal events in the person's life—a death in the family, a new job, getting married or going through a divorce, and so forth. Dr. Holmes also discovered that even talking about disruptive events could produce changes in the person's physical functioning. Using this knowledge, he and psychologist Richard Rahe developed their Holmes-Rahe Scale for measuring the impact of various life events on the experience of stress and its negative impact on health. The scale, which measures from 0-100, is based on how much readjustment an individual needs following a stressful life event. At the top of this rating scale, at 100 stress points, was the death of a spouse. Divorce was scored at 75 points, marital separation at 65, imprisonment at 63, buying a house at 31 stress points, and so on, down the line. For many decades, the Holmes-Rahe Social Readjustment Rating Scale has been used by professional counselors, physicians, and private individuals, and it has been very helpful in understanding stress.

22. Relationships

Realize then: When there is love in the heart, there is beauty in the character.
When there is beauty in the character, there is harmony in the home.
When there is harmony in the home, there is order in the nation.
When there is order in the nation, there is peace in the world.
Surely, those who love and are loved, are the happiest,
healthiest, and most powerful beings in the world.

—J. EMMET FOX

The previous chapter briefly emphasized the importance of positive, nurturing relationships in maintaining good health. Certainly, the Golden Rules would not be complete without devoting a chapter to this very important issue.

By now you are familiar with the concept of minimum daily requirements for nutrients in maintaining physical health. But what about minimum daily requirements of affection, appreciation, gratitude, and praise? How long can you feel okay about yourself and know your worth in society without positive feedback from others? Health practitioners have long understood the importance of meaningful relationships in health maintenance. Being in love and being involved in loving, nurturing relationships are among the most significant factors in strengthening the immune system and increasing longevity. So it makes sense that feelings of rejection, isolation, and loneliness have the opposite effect.

Among the most important considerations in appreciating the spiritual aspects of relationships is to recognize and overcome the delusion that we are separate from each other. For a better understanding of this idea, I recommend you read *The Greatest Thing in the World* by Henry Drummund, and learn to apply Drummund's simple but magnificent concepts to your life. You can expect to see profound changes.

MARRIAGE

Perhaps you have heard this saying: "A woman marries a man believing he will change, and he doesn't. A man marries a woman believing she will never change, and she does." It's important to be sensitive to and tolerant of differences between genders, and you must cherish and nurture your differences as much as you do your similarities, as each plays a role in your life journey together. Remember, anything worth having is worth working for, and a healthy marriage—which can be important in maintaining your health—is certainly worth your best effort!

One of the greatest gifts you can give your spouse is vibrant health. Pay careful attention to grooming, personal hygiene, and physical appearance. Bad breath, body odor, dirty hair, smelly feet, and soiled underwear can cast a real damper on any relationship; it certainly takes the romance down a few notches. Under all circumstances, practice common courtesy. Think back to the days of your courtship, and treat your spouse as you did in those early days of romance. Finally, it takes two happy people to make a happy marriage, so each partner in the marriage needs to focus some energy on himself or herself. Finding the right person is important, of course, but being the right person is equally so. *Married for Better, Not Worse—The Fourteen Secrets to a Happy Marriage* by Gary and Joy Lundberg is an excellent book that can help you maintain a strong marriage if you already have one, or strengthen your bond with one another.

Raising Your Children

If you have children, remember that they, too, are your teachers, and you can expect to learn a great deal from them. Do your very best to provide an environment that nurtures your children's health in body, mind, and spirit. Active loving in this way is the most precious gift you can give them.

Understand that your children and their peers represent the future of the world. As humbling—even frightening—as this may sound, we must celebrate this fact, because every new generation of the human family brings a higher level of spiritual consciousness upon the earth. For this to be true, however, you must realize that the values and attitudes you hold sacred may have far less significance to your children. Parents need tolerance to understand those attitudes and behaviors of their children that may seem to be contradictory to their own personal beliefs and life practices. Think about it—if children had never questioned parental authority, humans would not have progressed beyond living in caves! Therefore, parents should encourage their children to be critical, discerning thinkers, and urge them to respectfully question authority, including their own authority and that of their teachers, community leaders, and government officials. It's the natural order of our existence.

In Western culture today, almost half of all children grow up in single-parent or blended-parent households, which poses great challenges for all concerned. Never before has there been a greater need for understanding and patience on the part of parents and their children. Communication and courtesy is of paramount importance. Children need to feel honored and respected, thus, they should be spoken with rather than spoken to. Showing such respect for them will earn the same respect from them. And, clearly, it's important to let children know they are cherished and loved if they are to grow up healthy in body, mind, and spirit. For small children to feel emotionally secure and physically safe, their home must be a haven from the external forces of the world. By providing positive early childhood experiences, parents can be assured that their children will develop into mature, healthy, well-balanced adults who can make positive contributions to the advancement of the human race.

Sometimes it's difficult to remember that you do not own your children. It is my belief that your children's souls have chosen you and your spouse or partner to become their vehicle into the physical world. This is an awesome concept and, if true, it makes us better able to appreciate the wonderful gifts children are to us.

Protecting Your Children

A great blight exists in our society. Currently, about 6.6 million Americans are incarcerated in prisons and jails, and there are millions more who are hospitalized or institutionalized in mental health facilities. After they have served their sentences or been released from mental health institutions, some of these individuals pose a serious predatory threat to our children. Worse still, many child molesters and kidnappers have never been caught, nor have they served time in prison, and so they remain in our midst. Parents must guard their children against becoming victims of abuse and abduction by child predators.

Protecting your children is, perhaps, more complicated than you might have thought. For example, if your child is signed up to spend a week at summer camp, have you done a routine background check on the adults who will serve as counselors and guides? Have you done the same for athletic coaches, babysitters, clergy, scout leaders, and specials-skills instructors, such as music teachers who provide private lessons? Furthermore, we are beyond the days when "Don't talk to strangers" was adequate to protect our children from predators. Do your children know what to say—or not say—to strangers? Even more challenging is helping your children to understand that the great majority of non-parental child abuse and abductions involve adults or older teenagers they know and trust. And there are many other important questions to consider, as well. Do you always know the whereabouts of your children? Do you know their friends? How well do you know and trust their friends' parents or stepparents? Are you casual about allowing your children to stay overnight at other people's homes? Parents need to ask themselves all of these questions and more in order to protect their children.

While it's very important to teach your children to have a healthy, trusting view of their world, they must also learn to listen to their inborn instincts and inner wisdom. For your own mental health, it's just as important for you as a parent to learn to trust these instincts. A parent's paranoia about every imaginable threat could be very destructive to a child's mature development and how she or he perceives the world. Of course, all parents would prefer to raise their children to live joyfully, believing that life is a beautiful, safe, and secure place. However, in our real world, parents must take preventive measures to protect their children in body, mind, and spirit. This can be a delicate balance. An excellent book for parents on this sensitive and emotionally challenging topic is Gavin DeBecker's *Protecting the Gift*. For additional information, visit the National Center for Missing and Exploited Children website at www.missingkids.com. The Jacob Wetterling Foundation also offers an assortment of helpful brochures and educational materials for parents who want to learn more about keeping their children safe. Just call 1-800-325-4673 or visit their website at www.jwf.org.

Parental Abuse

Approximately 95 percent of parents who abuse their children were victims of abuse when they were children. This tragic, vicious cycle affects the lives of millions of parents in our society and poses a serious threat to the health, safety, and well-being of the millions of children living in their homes. Abuse can take many forms—emotional, physical, sexual, spiritual, and verbal. If you believe that your parenting behaviors are placing your children at risk, please seek help immediately for their sake. Free, anonymous professional help is available through highly effective self-help groups, such as the National Exchange Club Centers for the Prevention of Child Abuse. With 110 centers located throughout the United States, and links to numerous other professional organizations with common objectives, the organization can help guide you in finding appropriate help for your needs. You'll find their website at www.preventchildabuse.com.

SEXUAL RELATIONSHIPS—SEXUAL HEALTH

There is a good deal of research documenting the health-enhancing and life-extending value of a healthy and active sex life between caring and loving partners. In addition to its importance to procreation, almost no human function can compare with joyful and soul-satisfying sexual activity for rendering harmony within the body, mind, and spirit.

Because no other human act is so deeply tied to our emotions, it's somewhat understandable why so many of our artistic, cultural, entertainment, and social endeavors include sexually dominant themes. That being said, however, it's important to be aware of the damage that can result when we are continuously bombarded with sexual scenarios in the popular media. Every day, our economically driven media assails us with images of sexuality that cheapen the sanctity of meaningful sexual activity between two people who love each other. You can see, then, how the choices you make about what you watch, read, and listen to can positively or negatively influence your physical, emotional, and spiritual well-being.

As essential as being aware of overexposure to sexual images in the media is the need to perceive the more subtle signs of sexual abuse in any of its forms. In virtually all cases of sexual abuse, the perpetrator and the people on whom he or she preys experience the consequences of unchecked, inappropriate sexual expression and addiction. If you have been a victim of sexual abuse or you know that your behavior is abusive, I sincerely urge you to seek professional help. You have the rest of your life to experience the peace of mind and soul this will bring.

Sexually Transmitted Diseases

It's difficult to believe that an act as beautiful and sacred as that shared between two sexual partners can also have an ugly, even life-threatening side. Unfortunately, this is all too true. Sexually transmitted diseases (STDs) can be fatal, as in the case of AIDS; many others, while not fatal, are chronic, highly contagious, and resistant to treatment. Some STDs can cause infertility, and virtually all pose significant risks to intimate relationships and marriage. The most effective means of prevention is, of course, to totally avoid sexual contact with anyone you know who has an STD. Choose your sexual partners carefully and expect total candor and honesty about exposure to STDs from previous sexual encounters or other activities that can spread infection, such as the practice of sharing hypodermic needles among drug users. Encourage your partner to get tested for sexually transmitted diseases, and agree to testing yourself. Practice safe sex out of respect for yourself, your partner and the lives and health of any future children you may have.

FRIENDSHIP

No discussion of relationships would be complete without reflection on the wonder of deeply satisfying friendships. Each of your friends is a living, breathing gift of grace in your life, because nobody was ever meant to bear the full burden of life alone. True friends understand the principles of giving and sharing with humility and kindness; they show you how much they care for you without resorting to criticism or judgment (both good ways to lose your friends). A friend is someone who can provide thread for the holes you've worn in the fabric of your soul.

Do you have friends you are certain will support you in times of need? Do you count as your friends only those with whom you celebrate—share a few drinks, a hearty laugh, and a story or two? Do your friends evaporate like the morning dew when the heat comes on? Do you have at least one friend who would provide shelter if you were homeless, food if you were hungry, clothes if yours were worn, or a shoulder to cry on when you need one desperately? Through sad times and glad times, steady, level-headed friends are special people who can help you find your way through the maze and confusion you may encounter in your life. In other words, a true friend is someone who knows everything about you and loves you anyway.

A Friend in Need . . .

Surely you've heard that old cliché, "A friend in need is a friend indeed." But have you ever noticed how the saying is open to interpretation because it's not clear exactly who is "in need"? Think about a time when you needed help and you were willing to seek assistance from almost any source—even strangers. When you received aid in your time of need, you were no doubt very grateful and eager to somehow repay the kindness. Indeed, until you had the opportunity to return the kindness, you may even have felt somewhat uneasy. More than likely, you felt somewhat better when you heard of another person in need, and answered the call. Why? Because you became the friend who was able to give something of yourself to help another, and that was a deeply enriching experience. If you want to recapture this soul-satisfying feeling, make a conscious effort to be more aware of the needs of others, friends and strangers alike. Through sharing and caring with the right attitude, yours will be the larger reward. And it's an excellent way to stay best friends with the person in your mirror!

To Have Many Friends, Be a Friend

How do you measure up as a friend? Can others count on you during their times of difficulty and pain? Do you practice those qualities others can look to with confidence and impartiality when they are in need? For many people, maintaining true friendships can seem quite demanding, because every spare moment is filled with the activities, obligations, and stresses of everyday life. However, your life will be greatly enriched and you will find that your health in body, mind, and spirit will benefit greatly if you are of meaningful service, kindness, and genuine friendship to others. Almost everyone has the gift of compassion for others to some extent. Remember that "compassion" is a term that can be used to express the intense feelings associated with various trying experiences shared by those who have a common passion. This type of compassion is often learned from having already walked a similar path and stumbled over those same stones. For anybody who has experienced a very deep loss, often only someone who has spent the same agonizing hours, days, and weeks of sadness and sorrow can fully understand what that person is going through. This is undoubtedly one of the reasons why many people find their deepest friendships grow out of periods of grief and loss. Not surprisingly, when you have been down and out, the concept of true friendship becomes sacred and meaningful beyond description. Assuming you have had your share of stubbed toes, rude awakenings, and bumps on the head, isn't it good to realize that these trials helped you develop strong, fulfilling relationships with others? Considering the importance of friendships to your physical, emotional, and spiritual well-being, the following checklist can help you make and keep true friends in your life. On the positive side, ask yourself, "In my cultivation of friendships and positive human relationships, do I . . . ":

Express sincere congratulations to those who have recently been cited for a noteworthy personal accomplishment, in spite of any jealousy I may have felt?

Send a card, message, or memorial to those who have recently lost a loved one?

Write, telephone, or visit someone who is ill or injured?

Really listen when someone is sharing something from her or his heart?

Hold in confidence what is shared, if that is expected?

Remember birthdays, anniversaries, and other special days?

Give those whom I meet my best handshake and my best smile?

Make direct, face-to-face eye contact with others?

Show keen interest in the ideas and values of others?

Yield the center of attention to others equally deserving?

Generously extend praise and seldom impart criticism?

Provide accurate, detailed instructions and directions when needed?

Extend common courtesy to others?

Return RSVPs promptly and accurately?

Drive safely and courteously?

Learn from my social errors?

Keep my word in business transactions?

Make myself happier by helping others to be happy?

Pay my bills on time?

Show appropriate respect for people in public service?

Show in-depth kindness to children and animals?

Share what I have with those less fortunate?

Do my share of the housework?

Demonstrate total honesty with all people in all business dealings?

Express gratitude and respect for parents, siblings, and family?

Use discernment and question authority respectfully?

Pay my own way so I am not a financial burden to others?

Keep my voice low in public places?

Keep my appointments?

Arrive on time for work, social, and family obligations?

Avoid violence in thought, word, and deed?

Volunteer some of my spare time for deserving causes?

Keep my promises in personal relationships?

Return phone calls, e-mails, and personal letters in a timely manner?

Avoid name-dropping to impress others?

Express genuine gratitude for kindness received from others?

Teach others mainly by providing a good example?

Treat my family members as courteously as I do total strangers?

Work for social justice, particularly for the less privileged?

Remain tolerant of the inadequacies and imperfections of others?

Practice safe sex?

Avoid addictive behaviors?

Deal with anger appropriately?

Recognize my limitations and know when to say no?

Respect my employer and provide an honest day's work?

Respect other people's boundaries and need for privacy?

Avoid inappropriate touching?

Pay genuine compliments to others when deserved?

Show gratitude to those providing services for me?

Retain a positive attitude through times of adversity?

Extend genuine trust to those who have earned it?

Choose my words thoughtfully, realizing cruel ones can never be taken back?

Remain humble during times of personal triumph?

Promptly return borrowed items in the same or better condition?

Avoid borrowing money from friends and family?

Remain cheerful, happy, interesting, and fun to be around?

Use my unique talents in positive and constructive ways?

Keep my living quarters and vehicles reasonably clean and orderly?

Have and show respect for gender equality?

See the glass half-full, as an optimist does?

Live assertively, knowing the difference between abrasive, aggressive, and assertive behaviors?

Live courageously, knowing the difference between courageous and reckless behaviors?

Exhibit kindness and caring to those who are physically, mentally, emotionally, or socially challenged?

Use diplomacy and courtesy when engaging in sensitive relationship issues?

Share time with family and friends?

Respect other people's tastes in art, literature, music, and theater?

See the beauty and majesty in the present moment?

Show compassion through understanding, forgiveness, and acceptance?

Sincerely accept deserved compliments and gifts extended by others?

See and appreciate beauty and grace in others beyond the physical?

Encourage and compliment the artistic, creative endeavors of others?

Include the views and opinions of others when assuming a leadership role?

Communicate effectively?

It's important, of course, to examine behaviors that you believe may not be beneficial to cultivating positive relationships with others. Therefore, it's also necessary to ask yourself, "In my interactions with others, do I . . . ":

Complain and nitpick about almost everything?

Try to buy the friendship and goodwill of others?

Expect more from others than I am willing to give in return?

Spread gossip?

Lie or mislead others for selfish reasons?

Show disregard for laws and rules promoted for the common good?

Offend with bad breath, body odor, inappropriate dress, or sloppy grooming?

Use alcohol and tobacco products irresponsibly and disrespectfully?

Leave clutter, debris, and messes for others to clean up?

Have analysis paralysis, blocking spontaneous joy with constant *buts* and *what ifs?*

Talk boisterously, using foul language and rude behavior?

Constantly try to convert others to my way of thinking?

Waste food, water, clothing, and other natural resources?

Complain about government and politics but fail to vote in elections?

Participate in activities and behaviors that pollute the earth?

Constantly brag about my accomplishments?

Consider some people inferior and undeserving of my attention and friendship?

Exasperate and frustrate others with my constant procrastination?

Weigh others down by always being emotionally needy?

Always need the last word on every topic?

Abuse my body and my health so that, at some point, I will be a burden to others?

Overstay my welcome by remaining a guest in another person's home too long?

Feel bitter and resentful, and constantly share these negative feelings with others?

Make racist comments and tell jokes reflecting prejudices?

Obsess about personal appearance?

Have sloppy handwriting that is difficult for others to read?

Offend with disrespectful table manners?

Provoke fights by always having to get even?

Always see the glass as a pessimist would, half-empty?

Justify intolerance, stubbornness, and rigidity under the guise of principles?

Give up easily after only a mediocre effort?

Place more emphasis on wants than on needs?

Spend countless hours jabbering on the phone?

Play the victim and expect pity?

Discourage others by citing reasons why something worthwhile cannot be accomplished?

Constantly moan and groan about past mistakes?

Show personal insecurity by constantly worrying, fretting, and stewing?

Speak negatively or critically about previous, failed personal relationships?

Ridicule or make jokes about the religious or spiritual beliefs and practices of others?

Constantly tell the same weary stories and jokes?

Continually remind others of their past mistakes, hurts, and errors in judgment?

Behave selfishly, placing my own interests, pleasure, and happiness above others?

Hog the phone or home computer, not sharing in a balanced way?

Interrupt others while they are conversing on the phone?

Play music so loud that it offends others, including neighbors?

Act nosey, expecting others to share every personal detail and fact?

Steal or carelessly damage property that belongs to others?

Use the friendship of others primarily for economic gain?

Show arrogance, disdain, and cynicism for almost everything?

Ridicule, demean, and humiliate others, especially in public?

Use profanity, vulgarity, or obscene language over the phone or in e-mails?

Receive cell phone calls in public places, such as libraries, houses of worship, restaurants, schools, or theaters?

Tailgate, recklessly change lanes, and intimidate other drivers when driving?

Almost never say "I'm sorry"?

Almost never admit any wrongdoing?

Regularly forget to say "thank you" and "excuse me"?

Lack restraint in eating, drinking, and consumption in general?

Telephone others during odd hours, mealtimes, or while they are likely to be sleeping?

Casually drop by the homes of others unannounced, without being invited?

Act rudely, hassle, or be demanding of clerks, waiters, and other service personnel?

Track mud and grease onto other people's clean carpets and floors?

Casually break professional appointments without notice of cancellation?

Misplace or lose important items, documents, records, and related information?

Threaten to, or bring, legal action against others over trivial matters?

Forget to flush home or public toilets after use?

Toss debris and garbage onto public roads and highways?

Rudely yell and scream hostilities at officials and coaches at athletic events?

Talk out loud during movies in the theater?

Demonstrate immaturity and poor judgment in personal decision making?

Carefully examining and paying attention to your attitudes and behaviors may not guarantee better friends and more positive relationships, but your awareness and application of the principles involved will hopefully be a positive experience in your life. The outcomes may surprise you.

Remain Graceful

Whatever you do, especially in your relationships, do it gracefully. Then those around you will think kindly of you, even if you are sometimes a real social klutz—as we all are at times. Here's a toast to deep and lasting friendships!

23. Common Sense

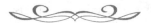

much human suffering results from events that could have been avoided had the application of common sense preceded the occurrence. The old saying, "Everyone has twenty-twenty hindsight" may be worth reflecting on as you proceed through this chapter. "If only I had . . . " is a common expression used by people who are feeling the remorse, guilt, and regret of not having exercised better judgment in matters relating to their personal health and safety and that of the people they love. The Golden Rules and themes outlined here can bring about a peace of mind that will help reduce stress, improve your health, and may even save your life.

AUTOMOTIVE AND VEHICULAR SAFETY

The statistics on automobile accidents are staggering. Are you aware that every fourteen seconds someone in the United States is injured in a traffic accident, and every twelve minutes someone is killed? Or that motor vehicle accidents are the leading cause of death between one and thirty-three years of age? That approximately 40,000 people are killed each year on American highways and that, among these, eight children are killed and another 900 injured every day? That the majority of all automobile crashes happen within twenty-five miles of home?

Every year, motor vehicle accidents dramatically change millions of lives, but practical strategies and common sense can prevent many of these tragedies and save countless lives. It should come as no surprise to learn that reckless speed and alcohol intoxication are the primary and predictable killers on the highway. But in addition to reducing your speed and not drinking and driving, the suggestions discussed here can help you keep yourself and your loved ones safe.

Seat Belts and Air Bags

Today, many people who use braces, crutches, walkers, or wheelchairs, or who are totally bedridden or living on life support, must do so because they did not buckle up. Protecting yourself against these kinds of injuries is as simple as putting on a seatbelt every time you get behind the wheel or are a passenger in a vehicle. When you are doing the driving, don't budge until all your passengers have buckled up—yourself included. Most automobiles are sold with standard front-seat airbags, which have saved many thousands of lives and prevented crippling injury and disability, so when you purchase your next vehicle, make sure airbags are part of the package. However, be aware that airbags can actually cause harm, as well, particularly for people who are unusually short in stature. Small children should be carefully secured in infant and toddler seats in the back seats of traditional passenger cars and SUVs. They must never ride as passengers in the front seat of any vehicle equipped with airbags.

Special Concern for Teenage Drivers

The National Safety Council and the National Highway Traffic Administration have released some alarming statistics on teenage driving: Teenage drivers are involved in automobile accidents more than any other age group; most teenage drivers do not use their seatbelts; compared with other age groups, more teenage drivers involved in accidents die; teenage drivers with teenage passengers use seat belts less than teenage drivers driving alone; teenage boys use seat belts less than teenage girls; teenage drivers of pickup trucks, SUVs, and vans use seat belts less than teenage drivers of cars; states with primary belt-use laws, where officers can stop drivers just because they are not buckled up, have higher teen seat-belt use, while states with secondary belt-use laws, where officers cannot stop drivers just because they are not buckled up, have lower rates of teen seat-belt use. The good news is that, from 1995 through 2000, an estimated 4,305 drivers aged sixteen to nineteen survived accidents because they were wearing seat belts.

As you can see, then, passing and enforcing more stringent seat-belt laws will save countless lives in this country. In addition, parents need to assume a very serious role in shaping the safety attitudes of young drivers in their households, and restrict the driving privileges—and perhaps other freedoms—of teens who refuse to comply.

Helmets

If you enjoy riding motorcycles, snowmobiles, or all-terrain vehicles, it is important to wear a properly fitted protective helmet that can minimize your risk of head injuries in the event of an accident. Passengers of these vehicles should also wear helmets for their safety.

Vehicle Maintenance

Carefully maintain vehicles that you and your loved ones drive. In particular, make it a habit to regularly inspect seatbelts, signal and hazard lights, headlights and tail lights, tires, and windshield wipers to ensure that they're in good working order, and remember to have your mechanic check the brakes and exhaust system annually or at the first sign of malfunction.

Keep Your Eyes on the Road

While driving any vehicle, do not engage in any activities that may divert your attention from the road, such as combing your hair, drinking hot coffee, putting on makeup, reading maps, smoking a cigarette or cigar, or talking on your cell phone. Just a split second could mean the difference between life and death for you, your passengers, and other drivers and even pedestrians. Do not drink alcohol or use drugs if you will be operating a vehicle—even some prescription and OTC drugs can cause drowsiness that may impair your driving. And always be aware that, even if your own driving behavior is 100-percent safe, the person driving the vehicle in front of you, behind you, or at the upcoming intersection may be 100 percent unsafe.

PROTECTIVE EQUIPMENT

Wearing protective gear and safety equipment when necessary applies whether you're at work for the day, at home doing chores or repair projects, or enjoying your favorite hobbies—not just when you're participating in dangerous sports or other activities. Protective gear includes gloves, hearing protection, helmets, machine guards, padding, safety glasses, shin guards, or eye protection when playing racquet sports. Also, it's important to be aware of others within your danger zone, especially children, who tend to exhibit sudden and unpredictable behavior.

FIRE AND ELECTRICAL HAZARDS

In terms of fire prevention, just a small investment of time and money can prevent enormous loss. Carefully inventory potential fire and electrical hazards in your home, at work, and in your vehicles. Make sure you have functioning fire extinguishers in key locations in your house—kitchen, furnace area, laundry room, workshop, and so forth—and install smoke detectors on every level of your home, near bedrooms, and in the basement. It's also crucial to have a plan for escape in the event of fire, and to practice your fire-escape plan with your family. Your local fire department can provide you and your family with an effective, user-friendly fire-escape and fire-safety plan. If you have small children, make sure your babysitters know where fire extinguishers are located and are familiar with your family's escape plan in case of an emergency.

CARBON MONOXIDE

Carbon monoxide is invisible, odorless, tasteless, and deadly. Early symptoms of exposure include disorientation, fatigue, headache, and nausea, which later progress to drowsiness, severe weakness, and unconsciousness. Sadly, within a relatively short time, carbon monoxide exposure can cause death.

The most common sources of carbon monoxide are natural-gas-burning appliances such as water heaters, gas-log fireplaces, kitchen ranges, and so forth. Also, running vehicles with gas-powered engines in enclosed, nonventilated spaces can quickly lead to a dangerous buildup of carbon monoxide that can be deadly. Fortunately, carbon monoxide detectors are readily available to help you be sure that the poisonous gas is not seeping into your home, garage, and workplace. You can purchase a carbon monoxide detector at any home improvement store. Finally, in many cases, employees of your local gas and electric power companies are available to check your home or business for dangerous levels of carbon monoxide.

SUNSHINE

These days, we are all aware that overexposure to sunshine can have some dangerous consequences, including the development of skin cancer. But did you know that some amount of sunlight is actually necessary to good health? In fact, adequate exposure to sunshine is crucial for the body's production of vitamin D, an important nutrient in bone formation that is essential to general health in adults and to growth in infants and children. Children who do not get enough sunlight are at risk of developing the most common form of rickets. Adults who are deficient in vitamin D may suffer from a condition called osteomalacia, or "soft bones," sometimes seen in older adults who do not spend time in the sun. Other conditions that can result from vitamin D deficiency are: bladder, breast, colorectal, ovarian, prostate, stomach, and uterine cancer, and all of the auto-immune diseases, including multiple sclerosis, rheumatoid arthritis, and type I diabetes.

Remember, however, that overexposure to sunlight still poses risks to health, especially for people with light complexions, red or blonde hair, or blue eyes. People who were often sunburned in their youth or who do outdoor work are more likely to develop skin cancer and, in some cases, a more aggressive and dangerous form of the disease known as melanoma. For people who want to get enough sunlight for good health but do not wish to risk negative health effects, it's wise to stay out of the sun after noon and into the early afternoon hours.

People who have greater amounts of the pigment melanin in their skin have darker complexions and, therefore, greater protection from the sun's ultraviolet rays. However, because a darker complexion means more protection from the sun, people who have darker skin need to spend more time out in the sunlight in order for their bodies to produce enough vitamin D for health. In fact, studies have shown that 42 percent of African-American women between the ages of fifteen and forty-nine were actually vitamin-D deficient by the end of winter. A very dark-skinned person may need fifty times as much sun as a light-skinned person to produce the same amount of vitamin D.

The pain of mild or moderate sunburn can be treated effectively with a cool shower or bath followed by the application of pure aloe vera gel, available in any drug or department store.

Heat Exhaustion, Heatstroke, and Sunstroke

Whether you're working or playing, you should always take precautions when you're outdoors in extreme temperatures, particularly when the humidity is also very high. Heat exhaustion is caused by excessive perspiration and dehydration, and symptoms include dizziness, headache, malaise, muscle aches and pains (particularly of the lower extremities), nausea, vomiting, and weakness. If heat exhaustion is not treated, it can develop into heatstroke, in which the body is unable to regulate internal temperature. Heatstroke is especially dangerous because it can result in major organ failure and death. Obese people are more vulnerable, as are those taking any prescription or illegal drugs.

Sunstroke is a type of heatstroke that results from prolonged exposure to the sun, in addition to extreme temperatures and high humidity. Symptoms of sunstroke can develop very quickly, including dizziness or faintness; sudden headache; nausea and vomiting; hot, dry skin; rapid heartbeat; and high body temperature. Without prompt medical treatment, symptoms may progress to disorientation and loss of consciousness and, if the condition worsens, death. For anyone who exhibits symptoms of heatstroke or sunstroke, immediate medical treatment is a must.

Fortunately, a few simple steps can help you prevent heat exhaustion, heatstroke, and sunstroke. Take extra precautions when the temperature exceeds 105°F and when the humidity exceeds 70. If you will be outdoors in these conditions, be sure to seek shade, drink plenty of pure water, and avoid products with alcohol and caffeine, which can dehydrate the body. To further protect against conditions resulting from heat and sun exposure, wear cool clothing; place cool, wet towels around the head, neck, armpits, and groin areas; and use ice packs, cool water-spray bottles, and fans to keep your body temperature down. Shading the area will also help prevent these conditions, and sunstroke as well.

LEARN TO RECOGNIZE AND TREAT SHOCK

Shock is the failure of organ systems and body functions that occurs when the heart and circulatory system are not able to pump enough blood to vital tissues and organs, due to sudden illness or severe injuries. Symptoms of shock include confusion; cool, clammy skin; weakness, dizziness, and a faint feeling; low blood pressure; nausea and vomiting; shallow, rapid breathing; excessive thirst; and weak but rapid pulse. Shock can result in loss of consciousness and death without immediate medical assistance, so if you believe someone around you is going into shock, call 911 immediately. While you wait for emergency assistance to arrive, help the person who is going into shock lie flat on his or her back and gently elevate the legs higher than the heart. It's important to note, however, that if there is injury to the head, neck, chest cavity, or spine, you should not move the person you are trying to help more than is necessary, so you should instead keep him or her lying flat with legs extended. If the person feels nauseated or begins to vomit, gently turn him or her to one side, with support for the neck if you suspect spinal injury. To the extent you can, try to control any bleeding, and keep the person's body temperature stable by providing warmth in cold conditions or helping the person stay cool in unusually hot conditions.

WHEN TO VISIT THE DOCTOR

At one time, health experts recommended that everyone have a yearly physical exam to stay healthy and prevent illness. Times have changed, however, and annual physicals are generally not considered necessary these days. Of course, visiting your doctor is still important in the prevention of disease and the maintenance of good health. Consider the following guidelines in deciding how often you and your loved ones should see the doctor:

- Infants and preschool children should have yearly physical exams.

- Women of childbearing age should have a Pap test and breast examination yearly. Concerning mammograms, holistic healthcare professionals caution against annual mammograms for women over the age of forty, since x-rays are known to be carcinogenic; however, many doctors do hold to this recommendation.

- Healthy males should have general physical examinations every ten years until about age fifty, and every five years thereafter.

- People with a history of heart disease or stroke in their family should have a physical to examine cardiovascular health every three to five years. People who smoke, have a high stress level, dislike their jobs, or lead sedentary lifestyles, as well as those who have elevated blood fats or high blood pressure, should also get a checkup every three to five years. Additionally, anyone who is planning to start a vigorous exercise program may benefit from a cardiac evaluation, including a cardiac stress test on a treadmill.

- All adults over the age of fifty should have a colon exam about every ten years, but more often—as advised by a doctor—if there is a family history of colon or colorectal cancer.

- People of all ages benefit from periodic oral cavity checkups and regular dental exams twice a year.

- Men who are fifty years of age or older should have lower colon and prostate exams every five years.

- Men and women forty years of age or older should have their blood pressure, weight, and serum cholesterol checked, as well as urinalysis and stool analysis, every five years.

- People who are obese, as well as people who have a family history of diabetes or hypoglycemia should have their blood sugar levels tested annually.

- Hearing and vision screening should be done periodically for people of all ages, and particularly for those who are noticing evidence of loss.

- Women who are no longer menstruating should have bone density exams every two years. Men should have the same test done every ten years.

The above suggestions follow the current guidelines of the conventional Western medical model of health care. For many, however, it would be well to consider visiting specially chosen alternative practitioners for prevention and wellness maintenance at reasonable intervals proportionate to your health status and personal needs.

BE AWARE OF ANIMALS

Never provoke animals that could bite or scratch you. Not only can broken-skin wounds become infected but, worse, there is also the danger of rabies and tetanus. Most pets and domestic animals have been vaccinated for rabies, but raccoons, skunks, foxes, and bats can carry rabies, and all precautions must be taken to avoid unnecessary contact with these animals, as untreated rabies can be fatal. Of course, if you have children, you must be sure to guard them against interactions with these animals, as well.

INVENTORY AND PROTECT THE CONTENTS OF YOUR MEDICINE CABINET

Until recently, Americans consumed seventy million Valium tablets every day. During the past few years Valium has been replaced by Prozac, Zoloft, Ascendin, and a variety of other prescribed and over-the-counter tranquilizers, uppers, downers, sleeping pills, and mood-altering chemicals. Statistics show that in the United States, every man, woman, and child uses eleven or more prescriptions for drugs of every imaginable variety every year. Many of these medications can be very dangerous if they are taken inappropriately, particularly by children and older people, so it's very important to safeguard your medicine cabinet to prevent children and older adults from reaching for prescriptions and OTC drugs that could cause great harm. You should also periodically inventory the contents of your medicine cabinet to discard any expired medications, and so that you have updated lists of medicines on hand in case you think some might be missing. Finally, you should keep the number for the poison control center prominently displayed near the phones in your house: 1-800-222-1222.

It's worth noting that the measures you take to keep the contents of your medicine cabinet out of the grasp of children and older adults can also be helpful in safeguarding your liquor cabinet to keep children and teens safe.

Keep a Poison Control Chart Handy

Keeping a poison control chart readily available is important not just for prescription and OTC drug overdose, but also in the case of ingestion of other poisons that are found in every household. Almost every product typically found around the house can be toxic if inhaled or swallowed, including fingernail polish remover, ink, liquid dishwasher soap, plant foods, rat poison, just to name a few. Therefore, it's important to prominently display a poison control chart inside the door of your medicine cabinet, near the phone, and in any other location that makes sense to you and is obvious to other members of your household.

Induced vomiting is a common and effective first-aid recommendation for some types of swallowed poisons, such as those listed above. An effective over-the-counter first-aid agent to have in your medicine cabinet is a syrup of Ipecac that induces vomiting. Carefully read the instructions before administering Ipecac, as this product should not be used for anyone in late stage pregnancy, older people, people with heart disease, very small children, or anyone under the influence of drugs or alcohol.

When other poisons, such as antifreeze, dishwasher detergent powder, furniture polish, gasoline, kerosene, oil-based paints, or oven cleaners are consumed, you should *not* induce vomiting. Instead, have the person you are trying to help drink water to dilute the effects of the poison and call 911 immediately for medical aid. If you are not sure whether or not to induce vomiting, or for further specific instructions before help arrives, call the poison control center at 1-800-222-1222. Each year, the poison control center gets 1,500,000 reports of accidental poison ingestion, most involving infants and children under twelve.

Finally, it's important to realize that inhaling the vapors of many toxic products is just as common as swallowing these kinds of poisons, and can be even more deadly. Also, many harmful chemicals that come in contact with the skin can be absorbed through it and spread throughout the body.

Using Over-the-Counter (OTC) Medications

Even though over-the-counter (OTC) medications are available without prescription, they can—and often do—have harmful and potentially fatal side effects if they are not taken with care. Between 16,000 and 20,000 people die each year from the inappropriate use of NSAIDs (non steroidal anti-inflammatory drugs) such as acetaminophen (Tylenol), aspirin, and ibuprofen (Motrin). The Food and Drug Administration (FDA) estimates that as many as 56,000 emergency room visits annually are due to overdoses of acetaminophen, with about one-fourth of these incidents being unintentional. And other OTC medicines may pose equally serious risks to your health. It can be easy to avoid these types of tragedies, however, and the following checklist can serve as a helpful guide:

- Consider OTC drugs and medicines to be as hazardous as prescription drugs, and take them carefully, as you would any prescription medication.

- Read the labels of all OTC medications very carefully before taking them, and use only as directed.

- Avoid self-medication for minor aches, pains, and illnesses.

- If you are taking any prescription drugs, ask your doctor about possible drug interactions or contraindications before you take any OTC medication. Even with the permission of your primary care physician, it's a good idea to get a second opinion from a holistically oriented pharmacist.

- Clearly and candidly inform your doctor regarding your use of any OTC medications.

Reconsider Your Attitude Toward Pain

While it may initially sound like nonsense to say that pain is actually your friend—and, in fact, something for which you should be grateful—take a moment to think about this. If a fire alarm went off in your workplace or home, you wouldn't cover it up with an armful of pillows and blankets so that you could no longer hear it, would you? If you did, you would eliminate the annoying sound, but the building would probably burn to the ground, threatening the lives of the people inside. Similarly, when a warning light comes on in the instrument panel of your car, you would not solve the problem by covering it up with a piece of duct tape. So it is with pain—it's your body's "fire alarm" or "warning light" indicating that something is wrong. Taking OTC medications may mask the problem, but are you really listening to what the pain is trying to tell you?

Unfortunately, some disease conditions are well advanced before any warning pains are felt to indicate that there is a problem. For example, about 20 percent of people who have fatal heart attacks never reported any previous angina, chest pain, or shortness of breath. This can also be true for other serious conditions, such as advanced hardening of the arteries, diabetes, high blood pressure, and lung cancer. From this point of view, when you experience pain, shouldn't you be grateful to know that your nervous system is looking out for your interests and reminding you that all is not right in your body, mind, or spirit? At that point, reaching for the convenient bottle of potentially dangerous pain-relieving pills that would only mask your symptoms might not be your best common-sense option.

LEARN CPR AND THE HEIMLICH MANEUVER

Emergency first aid classes are offered in almost every community. Your local Chamber of Commerce can provide you with contact information for organizations, clinics, and hospitals in your area that provide first aid training courses. I highly recommend that you learn how to administer emergency first aid—what you learn could help you save the life of a friend or family member.

Cardiopulmonary resuscitation, or CPR, is a combination of mouth-to-mouth respiration and chest compression that can help keep a person who has stopped breathing alive until additional treatment can be administered. First-responder emergency medical technicians (EMT), firefighters, and police personnel are trained to use CPR to save lives of people who have had heart attacks or suffered cardiac arrest for other reasons. Since heart attacks are among the most frequent emergencies to which medical personnel and police and fire officials respond, CPR is often used to describe this type of training. It's very important to note, however, that CPR should never be administered to people whose hearts are still beating, as this could actually cause significant harm.

The Heimlich maneuver is an emergency procedure used to prevent suffocation in a person whose airway is blocked by a piece of food or other object. Through a series of abdominal thrusts, air is forced up from the lungs and through the windpipe to dislodge the foreign object. While it's safe to perform this procedure on both adults and children, most experts do not recommend using it for infants less than one year old. Typically, the Heimlich maneuver is performed on a person in the upright position, but physical thrusts can also be delivered to a person who is lying on his or her back. This can be helpful if the person you are trying to help is too heavy to lift into a standing or semi-standing position and no one else is available to help you administer aid.

If you are in a situation in which CPR must be administered to a person who has been saved from drowning, it's important to first perform the Heimlich maneuver before moving on to mouth-to-mouth respiration and chest compressions. By first performing the Heimlich, you will be able force out any water that is in the airway, rather than pushing water further down into the lungs.

HANDLING AND SECURING FIREARMS AND OTHER WEAPONS

If you own firearms or other dangerous weapons, it is essential to store these items in a secure place in your home, out of the reach of children and teens, and to lock ammunition in a separate location in the house. *Never* leave weapons lying around in your home or on your property unattended. Young people who have demonstrated sufficient maturity that show an interest in firearms, *must* be given proper training in safe use and proper handling of these and other weapons.

CLEAN OUT YOUR REFRIGERATOR

Spoiled foods can make you sick, so check the freshness labels on all the foods in your home before you and your family eat them. Discard outdated foods and leftovers so that you or your family do not accidentally eat foods that are past their expiration or freshness date. Foods stored in a deep freeze for more than twelve to eighteen months should also be discarded.

AVOID BILLFOLD SCIATICA

You may find it difficult to believe that carrying your wallet in your back pocket can actually cause back and leg pain. This is because sitting for long periods of time in an uneven posture—due to a bulky billfold in one pocket—can gradually cause an imbalance in the muscles of the hips and buttocks that may, in turn, strain the ligaments and joints of your pelvic bones. It's especially important to remember to take your wallet out of your back pocket when you will be driving or riding in any motor vehicle, because the movement and vibrations may constrict circulation where the stress is, compounding the strain. Additionally, sitting in a lopsided posture puts pressure on your sciatic nerves, which extend from the lower spine and tailbone down through the buttocks and into the legs. Pressure on one or both sciatic nerves from sitting on your wallet can cause pain and weakness in one or both legs, sometimes referred to as "billfold sciatica." True sciatica is a condition that usually results from a ruptured or herniated disc in the lower spine compressing the root of the sciatic nerve. Symptoms include pain, weakness, and numbness of the affected leg and foot due to compression of the sciatic nerve.

TPK Leather Goods manufactures an innovative thin billfold called the TPK Mini-Wallet, which can hold up to twenty-four cards and twenty folding bills. The wallet is specially designed to be carried in the front pocket of men's trousers. For further information or to order a TPK Mini-Wallet, call 1-800-433-4653 or visit www.tpk-leather.com.

TRIPS, SLIPS, AND FALLS

Approximately 25 percent of all work-related injuries requiring time off for recovery result from trips, slips, and falls. The same kinds of accidents also occur in and around the home or during recreational activity, and are responsible for many thousands of injuries each year. These injuries may include contusions, dislocations, fractures, lacerations, sprains, and strains that can be serious.

Greasy, polished, icy, wet, and other slippery surfaces are often the culprits in slip-and-fall accidents. Likewise, objects that are out of place, strewn about, or unsecured—including hoses, litter, loose rugs on smooth surfaces, obstructions in stairs and walkways, power cords, and so forth—are significant factors in causing people to trip and fall. Obstructed visibility and inadequate lighting can also contribute to these kinds of accidents. You might think the majority of falls would be from heights, such as ladders, rooftops, scaffolding, and trees, but this is not the case. Nearly 90 percent of falls occur on a level surface or while descending stairs, so most of these unfortunate accidents can be prevented by keeping your house clear of clutter, avoiding slippery surfaces, using extra caution on ladders and stairs, and using reasonable caution when moving your body through space.

LIGHTNING

Worldwide, thousands of people are struck by lightning every year and, although lightning strikes are not always fatal, lightning kills more people than any other weather event. However, keeping yourself safe from this kind of tragedy can be as simple as taking a few extra precautions during thunderstorms. If you are indoors, do not take a bath or shower until you are certain the storm has passed; stay away from doors and windows; turn off and unplug appliances, television sets, and computers; and stay off the phone. If you are outdoors, stay away from water, avoid open spaces, and move to lower ground. Do not seek shelter under canopies, small picnic or rain shelters, or near trees, and stay away from metal fences or light poles. If you are able to, wait out the storm in a fully enclosed metal vehicle such as a car, truck, or van with the windows completely shut. .

MICROWAVE OVENS

Many holistically oriented practitioners discourage the use of microwave ovens for a variety of health reasons, including the suspicion that the microwave energy frequencies disrupt the electromagnetic nature of the foods being cooked. If you like the convenience of cooking food in a microwave oven, be sure you use only microwave-safe containers, and periodically inspect the insulation around the door. Cracked, frayed insulation can allow microwave frequencies to leak out that can be dangerous and destructive to tissue cells. If the insulation is showing signs of wear, speak with an appliance dealer who can help you order a replacement door from the manufacturer.

PROTECT YOUR PROPERTY

For peace of mind, it is important to reasonably protect your belongings—major possessions as well as smaller items of value. Since you do not want to become a target for thieves or those who would take advantage of you, causing you and your family severe economic and emotional distress, consider taking the following precautions to protect yourself and your loved ones:

- Secure your home and vehicles with appropriate locks and security systems.

- Do an inventory of your purse or wallet and make a photocopy of important items, such as your driver's license, social security card, and all credit cards, and place these copies in a secure location. That way, should someone steal your wallet or purse, you can immediately contact the appropriate authorities and promptly identify your valuables.

- Purchase an inexpensive home paper shredder to carefully dispose of unwanted documents with important information that thieves could utilize, such as old correspondence and bills from credit card companies. This small investment will be returned with the security of knowing that others will not have access to your valuable personal data.

- Finally, taking photos of your valued possessions can be helpful for retrieval and insurance purposes. These should be stored in your bank safe deposit box or another safe location away from your residence or business.

If your credit cards are stolen, contact the credit card companies themselves as soon as you are aware of the theft to report the items missing so you will not be liable for any fraudulent charges made to your account, and they can issue you a new card with a new number. You can also contact the three national credit-reporting organizations to report your loss so any company checking your credit will be informed that your information was recently stolen. The credit reporting agencies are: Equifax (1-800-535-6285) Experian (1-888-397-3742) and Trans Union (1-800-680-7289).

24. Ergonomics

ccording to the Occupational Safety and Health Administration, 1.8 million work-related musculoskeletal disorders are reported annually, resulting in over 100 million lost workdays, and a total of $116 billion lost to American businesses. The Bureau of Labor Statistics has found that twenty-five lost work days occur for every single case of carpal tunnel syndrome, a common wrist and forearm disorder often seen in clerical workers. There is much that can be done to prevent these and other work-related conditions, however, and this is the real objective of ergonomics.

Ergonomics is the study of the laws of work, specifically issues within the workplace that can contribute to stress and related health concerns. Applied ergonomics is the science that considers the relationship between people and their workplace and aims to improve comfort, well being, and efficiency on the job. Ergonomics includes the evaluation and study of all the various stress factors that could affect the physical, mental, and emotional health of workers; therefore, it is a complex field of study. Stress factors include the structure of your workstation, air quality and ventilation in the workplace, possible chemical hazards, temperature regulation, noise modulation, and even labor-management relations. Individuals in the field also research and develop safety communication systems, laborsaving mechanical devices, and personal protective equipment and clothing, and consider the shape and size of hand tools.

Taking note of the Golden Rules presented in this chapter will make for a happier work experience.

ERGONOMIC CONSIDERATIONS FOR THE SEATED WORKER

Approximately 70 percent of all work done in America today is performed seated at work stations. Since most of this work is done using computers, let's start with a look at the ergonomics of seated workers who spend most of their day seated in front of their computers. Ergonomists and practitioners involved in the diagnosis and treatment of the neuromusculoskeletal disorders in seated workers have long recognized the correlation between poor work posture and a variety of painful and disabling syndromes relating to the upper spine and neck. Among these conditions are: back pain; cluster, migraine, and tension headaches; elbow, forearm, shoulder, and wrist tendonitis; entrapment disorders of the wrist and hand, including carpal tunnel syndrome; neck stiffness, pain, and spasm; and thoracic outlet syndrome.

The Height and Position of Your Chair

Use a chair that provides comfort and support and fits your body contours properly. Most modern office chairs have been engineered to mechanically adjust to various body types. Carefully inspect your chair and take full advantage of all the adjustment features available.

Adjust the vertical height of your seat so that when you are sitting erect, your feet rest flat on the floor and your knees and ankles are flexed at ninety degrees. The depth of the seat should be such that, when you are seated fully upright with the small of your back firmly positioned against the lower back, or lumbar, support, it should extend forward far enough for you to place the width of three or four fingers behind your upper calf. This will help prevent the obstruction of blood and lymph circulation from your feet and lower limbs.

Adjust the vertical height of the lumbar support so it fits firmly into the small of your back. If the forward arc of your lower spine is either flat or average, most modern office chairs will provide adequate lower spinal support. However, if your lower spine has a deep forward curve, you will need a thicker lumbar support cushion. To add padding to a flat support cushion, place a folded towel or an extra pillow between the small of your back and the lumbar support to enhance your comfort. Or you may wish to purchase a commercial lumbar cushion from a medical supply store. These commercial cushions are portable and may also be used for additional lumbar support while driving in your car.

Armrests can be very valuable in helping you to improve your posture at work. If you currently do not have armrests on your office chair, you may wish to request the purchase of a new chair with armrests.

The Height of Your Desk

The top of your desk should be about two inches lower than level with your forearms and wrists when you are sitting fully upright in your chair with your elbows flexed at ninety degrees. Your upper arms should remain relaxed and parallel with the upper part of your body. If you are unusually tall or unusually short, you may have to adjust the height of the legs on your desk, and doing so may require some creativity.

The Position of Your Monitor and Screen

You monitor should be positioned approximately at arms length from where you are seated, and the upper portion of the screen should be at eye level when you are sitting fully upright. Tilt and rotate the monitor screen for optimal postural comfort and to eliminate reflected glare. If mechanical vertical adjustment is not available and the monitor is too low, you may wish to prop the monitor on a sturdy, stable object that will accommodate its best position.

The Position of Your Keyboard

As mentioned above, when you sit facing your computer monitor, your upper arms should remain relaxed in a vertical position parallel with the upper part of your body. Keeping your wrists pointing straight forward, flex your lower arms so that your elbows are bent at approximately ninety degrees—picture the letter L—directly in front of your body. The computer keyboard should be positioned just below your wrists and hands, not to exceed the reach of your fingertips when your elbows are bent at ninety degrees. Many modern desks designed for computer users have an adjustable keyboard holder that slides forward and backward, as well as up and down, and you will want to take advantage of this feature if it's available to you. Cushioned wrist rests are also available and can be very helpful in maintaining posture and increasing your comfort level, particularly if you spend many hours a day at your computer.

Conservation of Energy

Approximately 70 to 80 percent of human energy is expended in the maintenance of the body's mass in space and the movement of the body's mass through space. As a survival mechanism, we have an innate desire to conserve energy, and the least amount of energy is expended when the body's mass is maintained in a balanced position over its base of support. Anthropometrics, which is the measurement of body parts, has estimated the weight of the human head at between eight and fourteen pounds. The support structures for maintaining the head's position in space during movement or stationary postures are the spinal vertebrae and the discs, an intricate network of cartilage, joint capsules, ligaments, and numerous pairs of counterbalancing muscles in the front and back, and on either side of the spine.

Optimal Work Posture—The Comfort Zone

When seated, the position of the head is best in a neutral posture, meaning that the head is centered over the midline of the body when viewed from either the front-to-back or side planes, or with a slight, normal forward lean of about five degrees. Static work postures that require the head to shift away from the neutral posture—forward, backward, tilted, or rotated to either side—result in an unbalanced, asymmetrical load on the muscles. When this kind of strain on the muscles is repeatedly experienced for prolonged periods, it causes a buildup of toxic waste products in the muscles, resulting in fatigue and loss of efficiency. In addition, poor work posture produces asymmetrical compression on the spinal discs, and excessive stress on the supportive ligaments and joint capsules.

The neutral posture expends the least energy and results in the least amount of structural stress and related fatigue. This position also helps preserve the normal forward curve of the neck vertebrae. The four counterbalancing front-to-back curves of the spinal column are all designed to absorb shock and reduce structural and gravitational stress on the spine, which serves to protect the brain, spinal cord, and attached network of spinal nerves and their functions.

PREVENTING EYE STRAIN

Room Lighting

Your computer monitor should be the brightest object in the room. Dimming overhead lights will reduce glare and help prevent eye strain. Incandescent lights are preferred over florescent lights and, when aimed appropriately to illuminate your work, they will also help reduce eye strain.

To adjust your computer screen's brightness to the proper level, begin by reducing the level of brightness so that you have to strain just slightly to read the text on the screen. Then turn the brightness up to where the light looks and feels soft on your eyes.

Reducing Screen Glare

Position your monitor to eliminate any possible reflected glare from nearby glass pictures, mirrors, overhead lights, windows, and other sources. White or light-colored blouses and shirts result in more glare on the screen, so it's helpful to wear dark clothing when you are working on the computer. If glare continues to be an issue, use a high quality anti-glare filter on your screen. To help reduce the strain on your eyes, look away from your screen every ten minutes or so and focus on a distant object.

Use a Reference Material Copy Holder

If you use a side attached copy holder, adjust its position so the reference material is at the same vertical eye level as your monitor, just off to the side of the screen. For work assignments that require you to refer to the material for prolonged periods, it's best to move the side-mounted copy holder from one side of the monitor screen to the opposite side on alternate days, which will help balance the load on your neck muscles. Some seated workers prefer a center-mounted copy holder positioned at a comfortable angle between the keyboard and the monitor. This is a good solution to turning your head from side to side, but remember to follow the text with your eyes, rather than moving your neck and head, to minimize fatigue on your upper spinal muscles.

Computer Operators with Eyeglasses

If you wear eyeglasses, be sure they are the correct lenses for your distance from the monitor screen. If necessary, move your screen farther away from you to help compensate for your current lenses and reduce eye strain, fatigue, and headache. If you wear bifocals, it's important to ask your eye doctor about wearing glasses without bifocals that you can use at your computer workstation.

Simple Eye Exercises

Every ten minutes or so, take a moment to look to your right, then left, then up, then down. Repeat several times. Close your eyes tightly for a second or two and let them relax while still closed. Darkness rests your eye and the surrounding facial muscles. Periodically (if you are not wearing eye makeup) close your hand into a fist and, with your folded pointer finger and adjacent knuckle, deeply massage your closed eye. Don't worry, your eyes are not that fragile and the effect will be very soothing.

GENERAL CONSIDERATIONS

Take Frequent Breaks

It's not a good idea to remain in any one position for very long, because sitting still causes what is known as static loading of muscles, which produces toxic waste products and results in fatigue. Simple movement and stretching helps the body get rid of these end products of muscle metabolism. Therefore, it's wise to take at least a two-minute break from your computer every half-hour to get up and walk around a bit. Stretch and flex your fingers, wrists, elbows, shoulders, neck, and upper and lower back. Take mini-breaks even more often by doing some deep breathing; rolling your shoulders, neck, and head; and trying a few simple stretches, such as arching your lower spine forward and backward, and gently stretching from side to side.

Lifestyle and Nutrition

In addition to the postural, stretching, and eyestrain issues addressed in this chapter, you will remain much more comfortable and have fewer aches and pains if you adequately hydrate your body by substituting water for diuretic beverages such as coffee, iced tea, and soft drinks. You will have more energy for evening fun and play if you avoid gooey sweet rolls, chocolate chip cookies, and other starchy treats and eat your favorite fresh fruit instead. You will experience less swelling of your ankles and feet if you avoid salty snacks such as potato chips and pretzels and enjoy a banana or orange instead. Obtaining adequate amounts of calcium and magnesium in your diet or through supplementation will help prevent fatigue, knotted muscles, and afternoon tension headaches. In fact, due respect for all the lifestyle and health maintenance suggestions throughout this book can greatly assist in minimizing workplace discomfort.

Innovative Seating Concept:
The Stance Angle Chair and Plasma$_2$ System

One of the most exciting and innovative concepts in chair design and seating support is the Stance Angle Chair and Plasma$_2$ Monitor and Keyboard Positioning Unit. This system of seating includes a specially engineered chair and desktop device that gives the keyboard and monitor a vertical height adjustment that is always compatible with the desired posture of the worker. This unique invention, manufactured by HealthPostures, is a body-support system that allows an infinite range of postures, from the traditional sitting upright, to forward tilt, semi-kneeling, or reclined standing. The Stance Angle Chair and Plasma$_2$ Unit is truly evolutionary in its design and will play a significant role in solving the dilemma of stress from prolonged static postures for seated workers. For further information and illustrations, visit these websites: www.health postures.com and www.plasma2system.com.

ERGONOMICS OVERVIEW

The above information should give you a better understanding of the role ergonomics has in helping you stay well. Regardless of the kind of work you do, it's important to become educated as to how the design or layout of your workstation or work environment could be causing or aggravating back pain, headaches, or stiff neck. In addition, even such temporarily disabling conditions as carpal tunnel syndrome of the wrist and hand, or tendonitis of the elbow, are often the result of a poorly designed workstation that leads to excessive fatigue and repetitive strain to these sensitive tissues.

Stay Informed

Formal training on topics relating to ergonomics may be offered by your employer, local safety council, or community agencies. Ask to become a member of your health, wellness, safety, and ergonomics committee at work. Also, you will find that there are many holistic healthcare providers who focus on body structure and comfort in relation to overall health, such as doctors of chiropractic and osteopathy, as well as physical therapists and occupational therapists. Any of these professionals can provide helpful advice—all you need to do is ask. The International Academy of Chiropractic Occupational Health Consultants (IACOHC) provides resources for individuals and corporations interested in applied ergonomics at www.IACOHC.com. For scientific references focusing on ergonomics, you may wish to look into National Institute for Occupational Safety and Health (NIOSH) at www.cdc.gov/niosh.

Workers who are primarily sedentary will greatly benefit from information provided in *Sitting on the Job* by Scott Donkin, D.C. This book offers a treasury of insights and suggestions for people who spend their work hours in a seated posture. Dr. Donkin and his co-author, Dr. Gérard Meyer, have also written *Peak Performance Body & Mind,* which tells how to optimize the condition of your body to increase your resistance to injury and fatigue, and gives helpful advice on healthy living, emphasizing ergonomic awareness of the body's structure and function throughout.

Another excellent resource for ergonomic home and office computer applications is Ergotron, Inc. This award-winning company manufactures a broad, innovative line of ergonomic computer equipment that is used in design, desktop publishing, engineering, home, manufacturing, medical, and networking applications. Call their toll-free number, 1-800-888-8458, or visit their website at: www.ergotron.com.

25. Your Attitudes and Belief Systems

This final Golden Rule considers the importance of your attitudes and beliefs.

Much of your pain is self-chosen. It is the bitter potion by which the physician within you heals your sick self. Therefore, trust the physician, and drink his remedy in silence and tranquility: For his hand, though heavy and hard, is guided by the tender hand of the Unseen. And the cup he brings, though it burn your lips, has been fashioned of the clay which the Potter has moistened with His own sacred tears.

—KAHLIL GIBRAN, THE PROPHET

GUARD YOUR THOUGHTS

"Be careful what you think about, for what you think about you will attract."

"Whatever you label something, it will become."

"If you claim an impediment, it is yours."

"Fear not, for your fears shall be realized."

"As a man thinketh and believeth in his heart, so it shall be."

"What you think about and dwell upon will come into your life."

You may recognize these familiar sayings, all on the same theme and all offering valuable advice. The central message of each is to pay careful attention to your thoughts. Prayer must also be included when we focus on our thoughts, because it can be a powerful form of thought energy. For many people, the natural inclination during prayer is to focus on problems. Doing so, however, tends to magnify these issues rather than reducing them. As such, in our thoughts and prayers, it is best to focus instead on gratitude for what you have, and not let anxiety, fear, guilt, or worry about our problems get in the way.

This is my favorite prayer:

I give praise and thanksgiving for all the circumstances in my life.
I am thankful for all the beauty, love, harmony,
blessings, abundance, prosperity, health, wealth,
happiness, and wisdom existing in my life. Amen.

There is the story of a seeker who consulted a very wise old man about the solution to a problem. Upon reflection, the ancient sage replied, "The solution to the problem is, there is no problem." Learn to think of every obstacle with which you struggle as an opportunity for growth or learning. In this context, I recommend *As a Man Thinketh* by James Allen. The following is a brief excerpt from his classic work:

"All that a man achieves, and all that he fails to achieve, is the direct result of his thoughts. In a justly ordered universe, where loss of equilibrium would mean total destruction, individual responsibility must be absolute. A man's weakness and strength are his own and not another man's. They are brought on by himself, never by another. His condition is his own and not another man's. His suffering and his joy are evolved from within. As he thinks, so he is, as he continues to think, so he remains."

Your own application of the simple but powerful principles expressed in Allen's work can change your life. It certainly helped change mine, and I know it has been of remarkable aid to countless other people who have heeded his counsel.

Never underestimate the power of prayer. There are numerous documented stories of groups who successfully prayed for the healing of someone ill. To better appreciate the scientific basis of benevolent thoughts extended to or for others, I recommend reading Dr. Larry Dossey's book *Healing Words, the Power of Prayer and the Practice of Medicine.*

The Power of Creative Visualization

The capacity of a disciplined mind is an absolutely awesome phenomenon. Your 30 billion brain cells routinely function far beyond the combined capabilities of all the world's most powerful computers. Nerve cells in the brain called neurons represent an example of the most complex network of connection possibilities in the known universe. Can you believe that there are millions, billions, and trillions of neural connections?

The human mind and brain has a remarkable capacity for imagination. To imagine means to create clear pictures in your mind's eye. Do you realize absolutely everything humans have created started out only as a picture in someone's mind? The Golden Gate Bridge, the Great Pyramids of Egypt, the Taj Mahal, Disney World, the ballpoint pen. Almost every material thing we take for granted in our daily lives began as a tiny electrical spark of energy that followed brain circuits similar in each of us, emitting a picture on the mind's own "silver screen." This ability to create clear images in the mind's eye, also known as the power to visualize, can be an incredible force for good in your life. This is what creative visualization is all about.

You may be familiar with the saying *What you think about and dwell upon comes into your life*. This expression has many variations from many sources because it is so fundamentally true. Without consciously realizing it, we think in pictures to process information: apple, boat, car, chair, frying pan—you'll notice that each word represents an image your brain recognizes and understands. This is what allows any writer to convey thoughts and information to you. The important concept to understand here is that whatever you repeatedly visualize and dwell upon—consciously or unconsciously—you begin to create. Can you see how positive creative visualization is important in the creation and preservation of health and wellness, peace and prosperity, freedom from stress, personal advancement in all aspects of life? Can you also see how visualizing negative ideas and outcomes has the potential to create disease and sickness or perpetuate war, violence, destruction, poverty, and human degradation? Can you now understand the dangers of worry and fear, and the hazards of dwelling on all the bad news you hear every day?

Consider for a moment what life would be like if each morning you picked up a newspaper containing only good news. Stories about all the good things people do. Columns telling of people who are caring, kind, loving, and thoughtful. Citations of individuals who look after their families and act as model citizens—people who recycle, pay their taxes, and pay their bills on time. You would read about millions of acts of charity and volunteer work by individuals, service and religious organizations, public schools, colleges, and universities. This list could go on and on. Have you noticed yet that there are far more good things taking place in the world than bad? Consider all the countries that are not at war. Reflect on all the people who have not been victims of crime or violence.

It is true we have crime, poverty, violence, war, and significant amounts of sadness in our midst. To ignore this reality would certainly be inappropriate and uncaring. However, disproportionately *dwelling* on the negatives in life will only result in your creative energies reproducing more negatives. It's a matter of mental discipline and keeping all things in a balanced perspective.

You May Choose Your Future

Learning the habit of positive, creative visualization can greatly benefit your health in body, mind, and spirit. Picture in your mind's eye a healthy, robust, powerful, vibrant, and vital you. See yourself only as a picture of radiant health and happiness, enjoying abundant prosperity. Practice this simple but powerful exercise many times each day. Let this image become your attitude. Do this consciously, with undistracted attention and intention, utilizing the limitless and boundless gift of your free will. The more realistically you can imagine your desired outcome, the more effective this process becomes. By holding to these powerful visual images, the creative genius residing within you will have no choice but to reproduce what you visualize. Pretty exciting future, wouldn't you agree?

GRATITUDE

Attain and maintain an attitude of gratitude for the blessings in your life. Remember the wise counsel of the philosopher Schopenhauer: "We seldom think of what we have, but rather what we lack. This tendency is one of the great tragedies on earth. It has probably resulted in more misery than all the wars and diseases in the history of man."

FORGIVENESS

Step out of the role of judge and reflect on the role of forgiveness in your life. Experience the peace of feeling forgiven by extending forgiveness to yourself, asking forgiveness of those people in your life you may have hurt, and granting forgiveness to others, especially those who have hurt you most deeply. Deal with guilt, regret, and remorse, and then resolve to move on with your life. Anger, bitterness, isolation, loneliness, and resentment are the choices most of us make, consciously or unconsciously, but these feelings and attitudes are toxic. To achieve and maintain excellent health, it's imperative to find room in your heart to forgive and feel forgiven.

LET GO OF ANGER

Some people believe there is a place in life for justified anger. This would be a

situation where the wrong done to a person is so grave, and so seemingly un-
forgivable, that the emotions of anger, bitterness, and resentment seem fully
justified. For example: A thirty-one-year-old woman goes to a doctor for her
unrelenting, disabling migraine headaches and a bleeding gastric ulcer. During
her medical history, which included a review of the sources of stress in her life,
she confides that for two years, between the ages of eleven and thirteen, she
was sexually molested repeatedly by her stepfather. She feels her mother knew
about it and did nothing. When discussing this confidentially in a professional
environment, her face and body language vividly express deep-seated anger and
resentment bordering on rage. It becomes apparent to the doctor that these profoundly disturbing emotions are central in the clinical management of her illness.

This woman may feel that her anger is justified, and that she is, in fact,
deserving of revenge. What she may not understand, however, is that her unconscious mind does not distinguish between justified anger or any other debilitating negative emotion that can seriously disrupt harmony within the body. Over
time, and with deep, soul-searching reflection that includes emotional and spiritual counseling, she may develop the understanding that all her anger, bitterness, and hatred have no effect whatsoever on the objects of these feelings, her
stepfather and mother. Though the process will doubtless be painful and challenging, she must find a place for forgiveness in her heart if she hopes to regain
her health. There's an old saying that those who believe in an "eye for an eye
and a tooth for a tooth" are advocating a sightless and toothless society. Simply
speaking, if you want your circumstances to change, you must change your
thoughts.

LIVE YOUR FAITH

It it generally true that the majority of people who acknowledge belief in a
higher power equate faith with the name of a religious practice. But if you have
found yourself disappointed or frustrated in finding spirituality, hope, and wisdom within an organized religion, you should know there can be something
more for you. Don't assume that your faith and whatever religion you practice
are one and the same, and that religion is the only outlet for your faith. It is not.
You can, instead, choose to live your faith as part of a spiritually based life—an
act that is potentially more fulfilling and one that can yield happiness and a deep
sense of inner peace.

Ask yourself this: "Does my religious practice enhance my faith and result in
a heightened state of mental and spiritual health? Or does my religious practice
bring forth feelings of condemnation, guilt, fear, and anxiety regarding my self-

worth, and result in harm to my health and well-being?" If the latter reflects your situation, you may wish to practice your faith and spirituality apart from organized religion. Doing so may lead you to greater self-knowledge and enable you to discover the warmth and light that reside deep within, helping you to develop vital, nourishing components of healthful living in body, mind, and spirit.

LIVE PRUDENTLY

Prudence means avoiding behaviors today that you may regret tomorrow. This sounds so simple, but its wisdom is profound.

STOP WHINING

Repeat after me: "Never again will I whine." Whining is the very best way to chase away friends and opportunities. Stop bellyaching, complaining, finding fault, groaning, moaning, and thumbsucking. Stop playing the role of victim. Nobody wants to be nominated for the Crybaby of the Year award. Yelling, screaming, and venting your feelings to a trusted friend from time to time can certainly relieve stress and sometimes can even be a healthy practice, but do so with discretion. Words spoken in anger and bitterness can never be retrieved. Even if you feel you have legitimate reasons to complain, resolve to discuss your concerns only with those you genuinely believe can help you. The key is to learn how to be assertive without being either abrasive or aggressive.

DON'T HURRY THROUGH LIFE

Many of us hurry through life with a sense of urgency. Reconsider your ideas about time. Remember your spirit, your soul—the real you—is infinite and exists in that place where time isn't real and, therefore, isn't measured. If you are late to work or miss an appointment once or twice a year, you'll find the world didn't come to an end. Not only that, you will be more likely to maintain a normal blood pressure, and your heart and the rest of your body will certainly last much longer. In the end, the direction in which you are headed is more important than the speed with which you get there.

CONSIDER MAKING A RETREAT

Do you often find yourself hurrying and scurrying to keep up with the pace you have set for your life? Are the circumstances in which you find yourself so stressful as to be almost dizzying? Do you sometimes feel the need to get away from it all? If the answer to these questions is "yes," you might consider making a retreat. A retreat is not the same as a vacation in that its primary purpose is to provide an opportunity for uninterrupted personal reflection and a quiet time alone to unwind and ponder your life's journey. Most people make a retreat to give focused attention to the personal and spiritual aspects of their existence. Numerous groups and organizations, usually spiritually oriented, offer structured and unstructured retreats that are often located in a quiet, relaxing setting that is conducive to listening to the soul and cleansing the spirit. A fulfilling retreat has a balancing, centering influence on the human psyche, and chances are you will return relaxed, refreshed, and renewed, imbued with a grateful attitude and a spirit of celebration. You may find the effect so profound that you elect to make an annual retreat, a decision that could greatly benefit your body, mind, and spirit.

LIVE ABUNDANTLY

The infinite bounty of nature is proof to us that there is more than enough of everything to go around. Realize that the best things in life are not things. Be grateful for what you have and be willing to share it—more of the same will come to you. If you don't have money to give, share some of what you find most precious in your life. Consider everything you give as seeds deposited in wonderfully rich soil, from which, given the right amount of nurturing, you will reap abundant yields. Remember, however, that whatever you have shared with others, good or bad, will be returned to you tenfold. This is not a casual equation, so carefully consider the consequences of all your thoughts and actions.

LIVE YOUR DREAMS

Dare to live your dreams. Remember the words of the great German philosopher, Goethe: "Whatever your dream, begin it. Boldness has genius, power and magic in it."

FIND PLEASURE IN YOUR LIFE

There is nothing wrong with pleasure as long it doesn't deplete your health and happiness. Instant gratification can lead to long-term regret and very serious health consequences. It is important to have and to enjoy your pleasures, but choose them wisely. As with most things in life, moderation is the key.

SELF-ESTEEM

When considering your successes or failures in life, you may believe your sense of happiness and fulfillment depends on what others think of you. Certainly, we all find great satisfaction in the praise, recognition, and gratitude we receive from people we admire. However, even more important to your feelings of success or failure is what *you* think of *yourself*. Your sense of competence, confidence, and positive self-worth is vital to your happiness, as is recognizing the importance of high self-esteem in maintaining good health and living a long and fruitful life.

REGARDLESS OF YOUR ILLNESS, IS YOUR ATTITUDE A FACTOR?

Throughout this book, you have read about the body's capacity to heal itself when it's provided with proper nutrients, uncontaminated fresh air, pure water, structural and neurological integrity, regular exercise, adequate rest, and moderate amounts of sunshine. Add to that list a healthy, positive, spirit-filled, trusting attitude and belief system that motivates you to overcome those all-too-common negative, self-destructive feelings.

It's a well-known fact that negative thoughts and attitudes can make you ill, while positive thoughts can help you achieve and maintain good health. Regardless of what you may believe is wrong with you, or whatever physical, mental, or spiritual conditions you suffer, your recovery will likely call for a careful, soul-searching look into your mirror. You might ask yourself these questions:

- To what degree could my illness be a symptom of self-pity?

- It's true I am ill, but could I also be ill in spirit?

- Do I understand what is meant by the term "martyr complex"?

- Do I assume my health and happiness is guaranteed?

- When I am ill, do I seek a disproportionate amount of attention?

- Do I feel that my problems and life challenges far outweigh those of people around me?

Before you are overcome by the idea that you have a terrible disease, you may wish to reflect on your attitude toward life. You may be absolutely amazed to discover the miraculous healing power of simply changing your attitude and putting your shoulder to the wheel of life.

DON'T COMPARE YOURSELF TO OTHERS

When you compare yourself to others, you may inaccurately perceive other people to be superior—sometimes far superior—to you. At the same time, you may believe some other people to be inferior to you. But do you find, in making all of these comparisons, that you are never satisfied with just being you? By comparing yourself—with all your wonderful, remarkable, miraculous, unique, special, one-of-a-kind qualities—to others, you are setting yourself up for failure. If you believe in your heart that you are somehow inferior to others, you will always fall short of those people who you feel are better, luckier, wealthier, more beautiful, or more fortunate than you. In addition, your arrogance toward those whom you have judged inferior to you will alienate your spirit and the joy that should rightfully be yours. As it is with your health, in all human relations, you will wear the cloth that you weave, and how comfortably it fits may be more up to you than you have perhaps realized.

RECOGNIZE THE BEAUTY OF LIFE

Embrace the fact the world is basically a beautiful place and you are 100 percent responsible for what happens in your life. As Shakespeare wrote, "All the world is a stage, and we are all actors on it." Within the holistic healthcare philosophy, not only are you an actor in your play, you are also the director and producer. Each of us is a co-creator of our own world and circumstances, and we must take responsibility for ourselves and our actions. The gifts of choice, free-will, attention, and intention are your magic wands to access all the creative energies of the universe. Simply speaking, you may choose love, or you may choose fear.

Once you fully understand the reality that you are not only at the center of your own universe, you *are* the center of your own universe, you will benefit from an incredible peace in your life. And from that moment on, you will know with total and absolute conviction that nothing really harmful can ever happen to you, and you will live the rest of your life without fear. Even when you die, the real you—your essence, your soul—is immortal and, therefore, will never die. Read *How to Stop Worrying and Start Living* by Dale Carnegie and you can begin to experience the joys of living without anxiety and fear.

RECONSIDER THE NOTION OF OWNERSHIP

Anxiety, fear, negative thinking, and worry are all based on the assumption of loss, and loss is based on the assumption of ownership. But the idea of ownership is really an illusion, as we own neither our bodies nor our souls. Nor do we actually own our houses or cars, our spouses or children—not even the shoes we wear! All are on temporary loan from the creative forces of the universe. Your birth certificate comes without a deed or a guarantee. That simple piece of paper, which serves as your passport for this short journey on earth, will eventually return to its origins to become part of another tree in the forest, just as our bones will one day become part of the earth. Detachment from ownership is a great liberator and a significant step in attaining inner peace.

LEARN TO LOVE YOUR BODY

Your body is the temple of your soul. During the time you inhabit this earth, you must revere your body and each of its parts. In your thoughts, take every opportunity to bless your body and all its capabilities. This is especially important if you are injured, or if you are ill and your body is not functioning well. You must love your body even if you do not perceive it as beautiful. If you truly appreciate your body's profound design and efficiency, you will come to realize it *is* beautiful, special beyond imagination, and uniquely yours. Just love your body and give thanks for it—and do it sooner rather than later.

Cindy's Story

At twenty-nine years old, Cindy was a very bright and attractive but unhappy and lonely single woman who came to me with a variety of health concerns, including constipation, debilitating headaches, gastritis, low-back pain, and menstrual problems. And these were just the primary symptoms she had checked on her health history questionnaire. In addition, she suffered from an extraordinarily disfiguring skin disorder that was quite conspicuous in its absence from the health questionnaire. She had a very severe case of adult acne that covered her face, neck, torso, upper limbs, and trunk.

It quickly became clear to me that, for Cindy, the acne was a very emotionally sensitive topic—one she did not wish to discuss. In keeping with the unspoken message she was sending me, I decided not to mention the matter. Instead, we began a program of care for her other health difficulties and, in a very short period of time, there was notable decrease in the frequency and severity of her headaches, and greatly improved bowel function. Her lower-back pain was significantly diminished and she reported improved digestion and less menstrual cramping.

It was obvious that we had developed a positive rapport and a trusting relationship, so after Cindy had expressed glowing gratitude for her improved health, I told her that her headaches, back pain, and other symptoms were all possibly the result of the various structural disturbances we had found in her body's framework. I also addressed the idea that, when the body's framework is burdened by significant structural stress, these factors can create interference in the nervous system. The nervous system is the primary regulator of all the body systems and this framework disturbance can have many other negative health consequences, including digestive disturbances and constipation. Then I expressed my belief that the severe acne she was exhibiting could also be a manifestation of these other disturbances. Embarrassed, she flushed and tearfully acknowledged that she had given up on her skin condition. She explained that, since her teenage years when she had originally developed this acne, she had consulted a total of eight different dermatologists (skin specialists) and that none of their treatments had made any significant difference. In relating this information, her disappointment, anger, and frustration were very evident.

I encouraged her to accompany me to a full-length mirror used to evaluate our patients' total body posture, and asked, "Cindy, when you look in the mirror and reflect on your skin, what do you feel?" Without a second's hesitation, she blurted out, "I hate my skin!" After she calmed herself and her sobbing decreased, I explained how our thoughts and attitudes can affect our body's function. I gave several examples, and she immediately grasped the mind/body/spirit concept I was putting forth. From that day on, Cindy began to lovingly nurture her body, including its wounded covering.

Through continued structural care and other holistic approaches, her health, including her previously very resistant skin condition, continued to greatly improve, and with it her physical appearance, her confidence, and her self-image. Several months later, she moved to a nearby city to embark on a satisfying new career. At Christmas, she came home to visit her parents and stopped by the office to express her gratitude and proudly introduce me to her young fiancé who was as handsome as she was pretty.

Madelon's Story

Madelon a forty-eight-year-old, twice-divorced mother of five, came to my office seeking treatment for unrelenting pain, weakness, and loss of function in her right arm. She had injured it three years earlier doing factory work, and had not returned to work since the injury because she found that all physical activity significantly aggravated her condition. Her family doctor had initially diagnosed her problem as a strain disorder caused by overuse and had treated her for several weeks with no improvement. He then referred her to an orthopedic surgeon specializing in upper extremity disorders. Following his assessment, which included special imaging and laboratory tests, she received extensive physical therapy, in conjunction with muscle relaxant and anti-inflammatory medications. Unfortunately, this effort provided no lasting improvement, either.

Since she was on full disability under workers' compensation, her employer's insurance carrier arranged to have her condition evaluated by another specialist, which resulted in another round of extensive tests and a regimen of care. Once again, there was no lasting relief.

For the next two and a half years, Madelon consulted a variety of doctors, including the physical medicine specialty team at a major hospital teaching clinic. By the time she arrived at our clinic, she had consulted eleven different doctors from a wide variety of specialties and healing disciplines, and reported that, in spite of all the care she had received, her condition had remained unchanged. She graded the pain as constant and severe, and as a result, she remained totally disabled.

As Madelon described her condition, it struck me that she kept referring to her right arm and related disability. Under most circumstances this would not seem unusual, as this had been the site of her injury and the primary presenting symptom. However, what was revealing to me was the fact that, in response to almost every question I asked, her reply included the words, "my right arm . . . ." She repeated this phrase so often it caught my attention and I counted her use of it approximately fifteen times.

As we progressed through Madelon's very involved medical history, I began asking her about her family, including her children. She

YOUR ATTITUDES AND BELIEF SYSTEMS

described each child briefly, including their ages and the occupations of the older children. She said that her youngest child, a daughter, was still living at home. I then asked if she had any grandchildren and she replied she had seven, including two small grandchildren, ages three and one, and they lived at home with her and their mother, who was Madelon's youngest daughter. When I inquired further, I learned the children's mother was sixteen years of age, unmarried, and a high-school dropout who had first become pregnant at age thirteen, and then had a second child at fifteen with a different father. I expressed concern that all the extra work of having a sixteen-year-old and her two small children living with her must be very stressful and a source of aggravation to her painful and disabling arm condition.

"Oh no, doctor, " Madelon replied, "they are no trouble at all. She's a big help. In fact, I could never get along without her. That girl is my right arm." After a thoughtful pause, I asked, "Your daughter is your right arm? Do you realize what you just told me?" She began to weep silently, and with this new understanding, she unfolded the incredible emotional pain she had felt when her thirteen-year-old daughter had become pregnant. She was heartbroken, she said, because this daughter had been a victim of incest by her own abusive, alcoholic former husband, the father of this girl, and it was he who had fathered Madelon's first grandchild.

After she regained her composure, I explained the powerful relationship between the mind and the body, and how prolonged, unrelenting stress and unresolved anger can result in a mental-health condition known as *somatoform* disorder. This condition is an example of conversion hysteria usually expressing itself as a severe, often disabling physical condition, with symptoms almost always manifesting in the bones, joints, muscles, and nerves of the body—in psychological terms, the body armor. I explained that since the disorder results from unresolved stress, it invariably *resists* any form of physical treatment, including surgery. I explained that such mental health disorders must be addressed primarily at the emotional and spiritual levels, and this may be why she had been unable to obtain relief from all the extensive treatments and physical care she had received.

I gave Madelon an in-depth explanation of holistic health care and explained that I would accept the management of her case only if she was interested and was willing to embrace a body/mind/spirit approach to her condition. She agreed, and through focused, interactive counseling, physical reactivation, lifestyle changes, and carefully planned structural care, she made steady improvement. About two months after this treatment began, Madelon was at last free of pain and able to return to work with a totally new outlook on life.

I hope the information contained in this book has given you helpful insights into the important interrelationship of the body, mind, and spirit. Thanks to the combined efforts of thousands in the healing professions, much progress has been made to ensure that it will remain a key component of healthcare practices in the foreseeable future.

Notable Quotes— Wise Instructions for Life

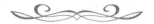

highly recommend *The Complete Life's Little Instruction Book* by H. Jackson Brown, Jr. (Rutledge Press, Nashville TN), an easy, pleasurable read that contains 1,560 simple, sage observations; power-filled lessons; and wonderful advice for more abundant living. This is a wonderful gift book for anyone, especially newlyweds, high school or college graduates, kids on their sixteenth birthday, or as a token of reward for dedicated employees. I would like to honor Mr. Brown's published legacy by sharing some of my favorite excerpts with you.

Choose your life's mate carefully. From this one decision will come ninety percent of all your happiness or misery.

Don't forget, a person's greatest emotional need is to feel appreciated.

Remember that a successful marriage depends on two things: finding the right person, and being the right person.

Judge your success by the degree you're enjoying peace, health and love.

Understand that happiness is not based on possessions, power, or prestige, but on relationships with people you love and respect.

Never compromise your integrity.

Don't be called out on strikes. You can't get to first base (or hit a home run) without swinging.

Remember that the person who steals an egg will steal a chicken.

Mind your own business.

When you need professional advice, get it from professionals, not your friends.

Share your knowledge. It's a way to achieve immortality.

Remember that what's right isn't always popular, and what's popular isn't always right.

Perform your job better than anyone else can. That's the best job security I know.

When lending money to people, be sure their character exceeds their collateral.

Remember that the best relationship is one where your love for each other is greater than your need for each other.

Don't discuss domestic problems at work.

Approach love and cooking with reckless abandon.

Worry makes for a hard pillow. When something's troubling you, before going to sleep, jot down three things you can do the next day to help solve the problem.

Be thankful you live in this great country.

Never say anything uncomplimentary about your spouse in the presence of your children.

Never forget that it takes only one person or one idea to change your life forever.

On your birthday, send your Mom a thank you card.

Be happy with what you have while working for what you want.

Never forget the debt you owe to all those who have come before you.

Don't be so open-minded that your brains fall out.

FINAL WORDS OF WISDOM

To laugh often and much; to win the respect of intelligent people and the affection of children; to earn the appreciation of honest critics and endure the betrayal of false friends; to appreciate beauty; to find the best in others; to leave the world a bit better; whether by a healthy child, a garden patch, or a redeemed social condition; to know even one life has breathed easier because you lived. This is to have succeeded.

ATTRIBUTED TO RALPH WALDO EMERSON

Conclusion

It's good to be concerned about your health, but don't dwell on it. Health in body, mind, and spirit is the natural order of things. The central theme of this book has been to share insights that may make you more aware that your health status is a matter of choice or a series of choices. Through the decisions you make, you create your own reality, and you should care enough about yourself to live by these commonsense suggestions presented throughout this book. They can profoundly affect your health and vitality, both now and long into your future.

What our country calls health care should, in most cases, be called disease management. For the most part, people wait until they are sick or injured and then go to doctors who must sometimes intervene with heroic lifesaving measures. At that point, the intervention is often very expensive and, in some cases, not particularly effective. In our culture, disease and injury management has become a trillion-dollar-a-year-plus enterprise. Only a small portion of that money is spent on practical and affordable prevention strategies. The purpose of this book is to help you make informed choices that will enable you to preserve your health and avoid the need for crisis-care, damage-control approaches to your well-being.

Having said that, it is probably best to remind you again not to become overwhelmed by the Golden Rules outlined in this book—they are not meant to be commands. Listen to your innate intelligence to make the right decisions and enjoy a lifetime of positive results. Some of you may feel you don't have time to incorporate the various health and wellness-enhancing suggestions offered throughout this book. But if you don't take the time to be well, you will eventually *have* to take the time to be sick.

Be kind to your mother earth, and remember that everything in the universe is interconnected. Modern man has probably done more damage to our environment in the past 100 years than all the world's inhabitants have in the previ-ous 100 million years. For the sake of your own health and that of your fellow beings, do your share to preserve our beautiful planet and its environment.

Be kind to yourself. The body is an absolutely magnificent creation—learn to love and cherish your body as a precious gift. Remember, however, that your body is only your temporary home, where your spirit dwells for this portion of eternity. Your spirit, the real you, existed before your body did and will survive after your body is no longer useful to you. By adopting this perspective, you can more gracefully accept the reality of growing older and eventually dying so your spirit can go on to the next level. Here's to your health, *in body, mind, and spirit!*

References

The following books are listed in the order they appear in this book.

Chapter 1

Carter-Scott, Cherie. *If Life Is a Game, These Are the Rules*. New York, NY: Broadway Books, Div. Bantam, Doubleday, Dell Publishing Group, Inc., 1998.

Bradley, Barrie. *10 Hidden Reasons You Are Sick—and What to Do about Them*. Becker, MN: Common Sense Wellness, Inc., 2001.

Chapter 2

Batmanghelidj, F. *Your Body's Many Cries for Water*. Falls Church, VA: Global Health Solutions, 1993. This book is available through bookstores or by calling 1-703-848-2333.

Chapter 3

Anderson, Robert, Anderson, Jean. *Stretching*. Bolinas, CA: Shelter Publications, Inc., 2000. U.S. distributor: Publishers Group West. Website: www.shelterpub.com.

Melnik, Michael. *Back in Step: The Road to Recovery from Back Pain*. Videotape, Prevention Plus Media Productions, Comprehensive Loss Management, Inc. Minneapolis, MN. Ph. 1-800-887-2282. Videotape and DVD. Website: www.preventionplusinc.com.

Chapter 4

Baroody, Theodore. *Alkalize or Die*. Wayneville, NC: Eclectic Press, 1991.

Chapter 5

Erasmus, Udo. *Fats That Heal, Fats That Kill*. Vancouver, CAN: Alive Books, 1987.

Bragg, Paul, Bragg, Patricia. *Apple Cider Vinegar—Miracle Health System*. Burbank, CA: Health Science Publishing, 1970.

Chapter 6

Howell, Edward. *Enzyme Nutrition*. New York, NY: Putnam Publishing Group, 1996.

Howell, Edward. *Food Enzymes for Health and Longevity*. Twin Lakes, WI: Lotus Press, 1994.

Lee, John. *What Your Doctor May Not Tell You about Menopause: The Breakthrough Book on Natural Progesterone*. Boston, MA: Warner Books, 1996.

Lee, John. *What Your Doctor May Not Tell You about Pre-Menopause, Balance Your Hormones and Your Life from Thirty to Fifty*. Boston, MA: Warner Books, 1999.

Posner, Trisha. *This is Not Your Mother's Menopause; One Woman's Natural Journey Through Change*. New York, NY: Random House, 2000.

Chapter 7

Sechrist, Elsie. *Dreams, Your Magic Mirror*. Virginia Beach, VA: ARE Press, 1995. The A.R.E. Bookstore's phone number is 1-800-723-1112, and their website is: www.arebookstore.com.

Fontana, David. *The Secret Language of Dreams: A Visual Key to Dreams and their Meanings*. London, England: Duncan Baird Publishers, Castele House, 1994.

Chapter 8

Leviton, Richard. *The Healthy Living Space*. Charlottesville, VA: Hampton Roads Publishers, 2001.

Chapter 9

Sehnert, Keith. *How to be Your Own Doctor—Sometimes*. New York, NY: Berkeley Publ. Group, 1986.

Valnet, Jean. *The Practice of Aromatherapy*. Rochester, VT: Healing Arts Press, 1990.

Chopra, Deepak. *Perfect Health—The Complete Mind/Body Guide*. New York, NY: Harmony Books, 1991.

Kapchuk, Ted. *The Web That Has No Weaver.* Chicago, IL: Congdon & Weed. Distributed by NTC/Contemporary Books, 1983.

Beinfield, Harriet, Korngold, Efram. *Between Heaven and Earth.* New York, NY: Ballantine Books, Div. Random House, 1991.

Redwood, Daniel, Ed. *Contemporary Chiropractic.* New York, NY: Churchill Livingstone, 1999.

Chapman-Smith, David. *The Chiropractic Profession.* W. Des Moines, IA: The NCMIC Group, Inc., 2000.

Breiner, Mark A. *Whole Body Dentistry.* Fairfield, CT: Quantum Health Press, LLC, 1999.

Huggins, Hal. *It's All in Your Head.* Garden City Park, NY: Avery Publishing Group, 1993.

Ziff, Sam. *Silver Dental Fillings—The Toxic Time Bomb.* Santa Fe, NM: Aurora Press, 1994.

Ewing, Dawn. *Let the Tooth Be Known.* Houston, TX: Holistic Health Alternatives, 1998.

Bonner, Michael. *The Oral Health Bible.* North Bergen, NJ: Basic Health Publications, 2003.

Ullman, Dana. *Discovering Homeopathy: Medicine for the 21st Century.* Berkeley, CA: North Atlantic Books, 1991.

Breggin, Peter R. *Toxic Psychiatry.* New York, NY: St. Martin's Press, 1994.

Breggin, Peter R., Breggin, Ginger Ross. *Talking Back to Prozac.* New York, NY: St. Martin's Press, 1994.

Breggin, Peter R., Breggin, Ginger Ross. *War Against Children.* New York, NY: St. Martin's Press, 1994.

Hawkins, David R., Pauling, Linus. *Orthomolecular Psychiatry.* New York, NY: W.H. Freeman and Co., 1973.

Chapter 10

Mendelsohn, Robert. *How to Raise a Healthy Child In Spite of Your Doctor.* New York, NY: Ballantine Books, 1985.

Mendelsohn, Robert. *Immunizations: The Terrible Risks Your Children Face That Your Doctor Won't Reveal.* Atlanta, GA: Second Opinion Publishers, Inc., 1993.

Romm, Aviva Jill. *Vaccinations*. Rochester, VT: Inner Traditions Intl., 2001.

Murphy, Jamie, White, Carol. *What Every Parent Should Know About Childhood Immunization*. Denver, CO: Royal Publications, 1993.

Cave, Stephanie, Mitchell, Deborah. *What Your Doctor May Not Tell You About Children's Vaccinations*. New York, NY: Warner Books, 2001.

Blaylock, Russell. *Excitotoxins: The Taste that Kills*. Albuquerque, NM: Health Press, 1997.

Chapter 11

McCully, Kilmer. *The Homocysteine Revolution*. New Canaan, CT. Keats Publ., 1999.

Ornish, Dean. *Dr. Dean Ornish's Program for Reversing Heart Disease*. New York, NY: Random House, 1990.

Dossey, Larry. *Space, Time and Medicine*. Boston, MA: Shambhala Publ., 1982.

Dossey, Larry. *Recovering the Soul*. New York, NY: Bantam, Doubleday, Dell Publ., 1990.

Chapter 12

Shames, R.L., Shames, Karilee Halo. *Thyroid Power—10 Steps to Total Health*. New York, NY: Harper Information, Div. HarperCollins Publ., 2001.

Chapter 13

Goldberg, Burton, Milne, Robert, More, Blake. *An Alternative Medicine Definitive Guide to Headaches*. Tiburon, CA: Future Medicine Publ., Inc., 1998.

Chapter 14

Schlosser, Eric. *Fast Food Nation*. New York, NY: Houghton Mifflin Co., 2001.

Fairburn, Chris. *Overcoming Binge Eating*. New York, NY: Guilford Books, 1995.

Fairburn, Chris, Brownell, Kelly (Eds). *Eating Disorders and Obesity: A Comprehensive Handbook,* New York, NY: Guilford Books, 2002.

Rankin, Howard. *Inspired to Lose*. Hilton Head, SC: Stepwise Press, 2001.

Hale, Lindsey, Ostroff, Martha. *Anorexia Nervosa: A Guide to Recovery*. Carlsbad, CA: Gurze Design & Books, 1998.

Chapter 16

Fink, John. *The Third Opinion*. New York, NY: Avery Group, Div. Penguin Putnam, Inc., 1997.

Epstein, Samuel. *The Politics of Cancer Revisited*. Hankins, NY: East Ridge Press, 1998. Website: www.preventcancer.com.

Diamond, W. John, Cowden, W. Lee, Goldberg, Burton. *An Alternative Medicine Definitive Guide to Cancer*. Tiburon, CA: Future Medicine Publ., Inc., 1997.

Clark, Hulda. *The Cure for All Cancers*. Chula Vista, CA: New Century Press, 1993.

Clark, Hulda. *The Cure for All Advanced Cancers*. Chula Vista, CA: New Century Press, 1999.

Chapter 19

Schmidt, Michael. *Smart Fats*. Berkeley, CA: Frog, Ltd., North Atlantic Books, 1997.

Chapter 20

Burr, Harold Saxton. *Blueprint for Immortality: The Electric Patterns of Life*. London, England: C. W. Daniel Publ., 1972 (reprinted 2000).

Becker, Robert. *The Body Electric*. New York, NY: William Morrow and Co. Inc., 1985.

Gerber, Richard. *Vibrational Medicine*. Rochester, VT: Inner Traditions Int'l., 1996.

Gerber, Richard. *A Practical Guide to Vibrational Medicine*. New York, NY: Quill, HarperCollins Publ., 2001.

Chopra, Deepak. *Quantum Healing*. New York, NY: Bantam, Doubleday, Dell, 1990.

McTaggart, Lynne. *The Field*. New York, NY: HarperCollins Publ., Inc., 2002.

Pert, Candace. *Molecules of Emotion*. New York, NY: Simon and Schuster, 1997.

Schmidt, Michael, Smith, Lendon H., Sehnert, Keith. *Beyond Antibiotics*. Berkeley, CA: North Atlantic Books, 1994.

Hiestand, Denie, Hiestand, Shelley. *Electrical Nutrition*. New York, NY: Avery, Penguin Putnam, Inc., 2001.

Chapter 21

Gibran, Kahlil. *The Prophet.* New York, NY: Random House, 1968.

Depree, Max. *The Art of Leadership.* New York, NY: Doubleday, Dell Publ. Group, Inc. 1990.

Tolle, Eckhart. *The Power of Now.* Novato, CA: New World Library, 1999.

Chapter 22

Drummond, Henry. *The Greatest Thing in the World.* London, England: Hodder and Stoughton Publ., 1880.

Lundberg, Gary, Lundberg, Joy. *Married for Better, Not for Worse—The Fourteen Secrets to a Happy Marriage.* New York, NY: Viking Press, 2001.

DeBecker, Gavin. *Protecting the Gift.* New York, NY: Dell Books, 2000.

Chapter 24

Donkin, Scott. *Sitting on the Job.* North Bergen, NJ: Basic Health Publ., 2002.

Donkin, Scott, Meyer, Gerard. *Peak Performance.* North Bergen, NJ: Basic Health Publ., 2002.

Chapter 25

Allen, James. *As a Man Thinketh.* New York, NY: Barnes and Noble Books, 1983.

Dossey, Larry. *Healing Words, the Power of Prayer and the Practice of Medicine.* New York, NY: HarperCollins Publ., 1995.

Carnegie, Dale. *How to Stop Worrying and Start Living.* New York, NY: Pocket Books, Simon & Schuster, 1948 (Reprinted 1984).

Conclusion

Brown, H. Jackson, Jr. *The Complete Life's Little Instruction Book.* Nashville, TN: Rutledge Hill Press, 2000.

Recommended Reading

These recommended books are complementary to the natural, holistic approach to health and wellness.

Brennen, Barbara Ann. *Hands of Light*. New York, NY: Bantam Books, 1993.

Buscaglia, Leo F. *Living, Loving and Learning*. New York, NY: Fawcett-Columbine Publ., 1990.

Epstein, Samuel S. *Unreasonable Risk: How to Avoid Cancer from Cosmetics and Personal Care Products—The Neways Story*. Chicago, IL: Environmental Toxicology, 2001.

Gould, M. *Staying Sober—Tips for Working a Twelve Step Program of Recovery*. Center City, MN: Hazeldon Press, 1999.

Gray, John. *Men, Women and Relationships: Making Peace with the Opposite Sex*. Hillsboro, OR: Beyond Words Publ., Inc., 2002.

Hawkins, David. *Power vs Force*. Carson, CA: Hay House Inc., 2002.

Hay, Louise L. *You Can Heal Your Life*. Carson, CA: Hay House, Inc., 1999.

Heimlich, Jane. *What Your Doctor Won't Tell You*. New York, NY: HarperCollins Publ., 1990.

Huggins, Hal. *Uninformed Consent*. Charlottesville, VA: Hampton Roads Publ., 1999.

Jarvis, D.C. *Folk Medicine*. New York, NY: Ballantine Fawcett Books, 1991.

Jensen, Bernard, Anderson, Mark. *Empty Harvest*. Garden City Park, NY: Avery Publ. Group Inc., 1993.

Kubler-Ross, Elisabeth. *On Death and Dying*. New York, NY: Collier Books, Macmillan Publ. Co., 1997.

Lark, Susan. *Premenstrual Syndrome Self-Help Book*. Los Altos, CA: PMS Self-Help Center, 1993.

Mitchell, Byron Katie. *Loving What Is—Four Questions That Can Change Your Life*. New York, NY: Three Rivers Press, Member of the Crown Publishing Group, a Division of Random House, 2002.

Murphy, Michael. *The Future of the Body*. New York, NY: The Putnam Publ. Group, 1993.

Potter-Efron, Ron, Potter-Efron, Pat. *Letting Go of Anger*. Oakland, CA: New Harbinger Publ., 1995.

Ray, Paul, Anderson, Sherry Ruth. *Cultural Creatives*. New York, NY: Crown Publ. Co., 2001.

Richardson, Cheryl. *Take Time for Your Life*. New York, NY: Broadway Books, 1999.

Shealy, C. Norman, Myss, Carolyn M. *The Creation of Health*. Walpole, NH: Stillpoint Publ., 1993.

Shield, B., Carlson, R. *For the Love of God*. Novato, CA: New World Library, 1990.

Steinman, David. *Diet for a Poisoned Planet*. New York, NY: Ballantine Books, 1990.

Sugrue, Thomas. *There Is a River*. Virginia Beach, VA: ARE Press, 1997.

Zukov, Gary. *The Seat of the Soul*. New York, NY: Simon and Schuster, 1990.

Zukov, Gary, Francis, Linda. *The Heart of the Soul*. New York, NY: Simon and Schuster, 2002.

Resources and Websites

Listed in order of appearance in the book.

Chapter 3

New Balance Athletic Shoe, Inc.
Brighton Landing, 20 Guest Street
Boston, MA 02135-2008
Ph: 1-800-253-7463 / 1-617-783-4000
Fax: 1-617-787-9355
Website: www.newbalance.com
e-mail:
    customer.service@newbalance.com

**Comprehensive Loss
  Management, Inc.**
15800 32nd Avenue North #106
Minneapolis, MN 55447
e-mail: plglynn@clmi-training.com
    (Paul Glynn is company spokesperson)
Website: www.clmi-training.com

Chapter 4

NuHealth Wellness
Website: www.nuhealthwellness.com

**Vaxa—Natural Solutions for
  Life's Challenges**
4010 W. State Street
Tampa, FL 33609

Ph: 1-877-622-8292
Fax: 1-888-734-4154
Website: www.Vaxa.com
e-mail: customerservice@vaxa.com

Chapter 6

Carlson Laboratories
15 College Drive
Arlington Heights, IL 60004-1985
Ph: 1-888-234-5656 / 1-847-255-1600
Fax: 1-847-255-1605
Website: www.carlsonlabs.com
e-mail: Carlson@carlsonlabs.com

Chapter 7

P.F. Pillows
Saint Paul, MN
Ph: 1-651-222-5868
Website: www.pfpillows.com
e-mail: PFP@PFPillows.com

Tempur-Pedic
1713 Jaggie Fox Way
Lexington, KY 40511
Ph: 1-800-821-6621
Fax: 1-859-514-5826
Website: www.tempurpedic.com
e-mail: info@tempurpedic.com

**American Academy of Sleep
  Medicine**
1 Westbrook Corporate Center,
  Suite 920
Westchester, IL 60154
Ph: 1-708-492-0930
Fax: 1-708-492-0943
Website: www.aasmnet.org

Chapter 8

Allernet
Website: www.allernet.com

Chapter 9

**American Chiropractic
  Association**
1701 Clarendon Boulevard
Arlington, VA 22209
Ph: 1-800-986-4636
Fax: 1-703-243-2593
Website: www.amerchiro.org
e-mail: info@amerchiro.org

**International Chiropractic
  Association**
1110 North Glebe Road
Arlington, VA 22201
Ph: 1-800-423-4690 / 1-703-528-5000
Fax: 1-703-528-5023
Website: www.chiropractic.org
e-mail: chiro@chiropractic.org

**North American Society of
  Homeopaths**
1122 East Pike Street #1122
Seattle, WA 98112
Ph: 1-206-720-7000
Fax: 1-208-248-1942

Website: www.homeopathy.org
E-mail: nashinfo@aol.com

The Holistic Dental Association
P.O. Box 5007
Durango, CO 81301
Fax: 1-970-259-1091
Website: www.holisticdental.org
e-mail: info@holisticdental.org

**American Holistic Health
  Association**
P.O. Box 17400
Anaheim, CA 92817-7400
Ph: 1-714-779-6152
Website: www.ahha.org
e-mail: mail@ahha.org

**American Holistic Medical
  Association**
12101 Menaul Blvd NE, Suite C
Albuquerque, NM 87112
Ph: 1-505-292-7788
Fax: 1-505-293-758
Website: www.holisticmedicine.org
e-mail: info@holisticmedicine.org

**American Holistic Nurses'
  Association**
P.O. Box 2130
Flagstaff, AZ 86003-2130
Ph: 1-800-278-2462
Fax: 1-928-526-2752
Website: www.ahna.org
e-mail: info@ahna.org

NuHealthWellness
Website:
  www.nuhealthwellness.com

Chapter 10

Narcotics Anonymous
PO Box 9999
Van Nuys, CA 91409
Ph: 1-818-773-9999
Fax: 1-818-700-0700
Website: www.na.org
e-mail: FSTeam@na.org

Al-Anon Family Group Headquarters, Inc.
1600 Corporate Landing Parkway
Virginia Beach, VA 23454-5617
Ph: 1-757-563-1600
Fax: 1-757-563-1655
Website: www.al-anon.alateen.org
e-mail: WSO@al-anon.org

The United Way—First Call for Help
701 North Fairfax Street
Alexandria, VA 22314
Ph: 1-703-836-7112
Fax: 1-703-683-7840
Website: www.unitedway.org

Centers for Disease Control— National Immunization Program
NIP Public Inquiries
Mailstop E-05
1600 Clifton Rd, NE
Atlanta, GA 30333
Ph: 1-800-232-2522 (Immunization Hotline)
Fax: 1-888-232-3299
Website: www.cdc.gov/nip
e-mail: nipinfo@cdc.gov

National Vaccine Information Center
421 E. Church Street
Vienna, VA 22180
Ph: 1-703-938-0342
Fax: 1-703-938-5768
Website: www.nvic.org

Poison Control Center
Ph:1-800-222-1222

American Dental Association (ADA)
211 East Chicago Avenue
Chicago, IL 60611-2678
Ph: 1-312-440-2500
Fax: 1-312-440-7494
Website: www.ada.org

The Fluoride Action Network
39 Green Street
Burlington, VT 05401
Ph: 1-802-859-3363
Fax: 1-315-379-0448
Website: www.fluoridealert.org
e-mail: info@flouridealert.org

The Agency for Toxic Substances and Disease Registry
Division of Toxicology
1600 Clifton Road NE
Mailstop E-29
Atlanta, GA 30333
Ph: 1-888-422-8737
Fax: 1-404-498-0093
Website: www.atsdr.cdc.gov
e-mail: atsdric@cdc.gov

Neways International
2089 West Neways Drive
Springville, UT 84663
Ph: 1-801-418-2000
Fax: 1-801-418-2195
e-mail: distributor_rel@neways.com
Website: www.neways.com

Chapter 11

National Stroke Association
9707 E. Easter Lane
Englewood, CO 80112
Ph: 1-800-787-6537 / 1-303-649-9299
Fax: 1-303-649-1328
Website: www.stroke.org.
e-mail: sgeris@stroke.org

Chapter 14

National Eating Disorders Association
Website:
www.nationaleatingdisorders.org

Overeaters Anonymous
Website:
www.overeatersanonymous.org

Chapter 15

Arthritis Foundation
1330 West Peachtree Street, NW
Atlanta, GA 30357-0669
Ph: 1-800-283-7800 (Option 5)
Fax: 1-204-480-4774
Website: www.arthritis.org
e-mail: help@arthritis.org

The Arthritis Trust of America
7376 Walker Road
Fairview, TN 37062-8141
Ph/Fax: 1-615-799-1002

Website: arthritistrust.org
e-mail: admin@arthritistrust.org

Graston Technique, div. Therapy Care Resources, Inc.
205 Worcester Court A5
Falmouth, MA 02540
Ph: 1-866-926-2828
Fax: 1-508-548-8813
Website: www.grastontechnique.com
e-mail: graston.information@graston
technique.com

Respondex • For information and practitioners, contact:

International Academy of Chiropractic Occupational Health Consultants (IACOHC)
930 Crestview Lane
Owatonna, MN 55060-2116
Ph: 1-507-455-1025
Fax: 1-507-455-0922
Website: www.IACOHC.com
e-mail: iacohc@mnic.net

Chapter 16

National Cancer Institute (NCI)
Cancer Information Service
6116 Executive Boulevard
Rockville, MD 20882
Ph: 1-800-422-6237
Fax: 1-301-402-0555
Website: www.cancer.gov

Life Source Basics
3388 Mike Collins Drive
Eagan, MN 55121
Ph: 1-877-346-6863 / 1-651-675-0146
Fax: 1-651-675-0400
Website: www.lifesourcebasics.com

Institute for the Study of Health and Illness at Commonweal
Rachel Naomi Remen, M.D.,
    Director
P.O. Box 316
Bolinas, CA 94924
Ph: 1-415-868-2642
Fax: 1-415-868-2230
Website:
    www.commonweal.org/ashi
e-mail: ishi@igc.org

Chapter 19

National Mental Health Awareness Campaign
Website: www.nostigma.org
e-mail: info@nostigma.org

Depression and Bipolar Support Alliance
730 N. Franklin Street, Suite 501
Chicago, IL 60610-7224
Ph: 1-800-826-3632
Fax: 1-312-642-7243
Website: www.dbsalliance.org
e-mail: infopack@dbsalliance.org

Chapter 22

National Center for Missing and Exploited Children
Charles B. Wang International
    Children's Building
699 Prince Street
Alexandria, VA 22314-3175
Ph: 1-800-843-5678 (Hotline)
Fax: 1-703-274-2200
Website: www.missingkids.com

Jacob Wetterling Foundation
33 Minnesota Street
PO Box 639
St. Joseph, MN 56374
Ph: 1-800-325-4673 / 1-320-363-0470
Fax: 1-320-363-0473
Website: www.jwf.org
e-mail: jacob@jwg.org

National Exchange Club Centers for the Prevention of Child Abuse
3050 Central Avenue
Toledo, OH 43606
Ph: 1-800-924-2643 / 1-419-535-3232
Fax: 1-419-535-1989
Website:
    www.preventchildabuse.com
e-mail:
    info@preventchildabuse.com

Chapter 23

TPK Leather Goods
316 Industrial Boulevard
Waconia, MN 55387
Ph: 1-800-433-4653
Fax: 1-952-442-4525
Website: www.tpk-leather.com
e-mail: sales@tpkgolf.com

Credit Reporting Agencies
Equifax: 1-800-535-6285
Experian: 1-888-397-3742
Trans Union: 1-800-680-7289

Chapter 24

Health Postures, Inc.
The Stance Angle Chair
and Plasma$_2$ System
100 East Main Street
Belle Plaine, MN 56011
Ph: 1-800-277-1841 / 1-952-873-3330
Fax: 1-952-873-3350
Website: www.healthpostures.com
Website: www.plasma2.com
e-mail: info@healthpostures.com

**International Academy of
Chiropractic Occupational
Health Consultants (IACOHC)**
Ph: 1-507-455-1025
Website: www.IACOHC.com
e-mail: iacohc@mnic.net

**National Institute for
Occupational Safety
and Health (NIOSH)**
4676 Columbia Parkway
Mail Stop C-13
Cincinnati, Ohio 45226
Ph: 1-800-356-4674
Fax: 1-513-533-8573
Website: www.cdc.gov/niosh
e-mail: pubstast@cdc.gov

Ergotron, Inc.
1181 Trapp Road
St. Paul, MN 55121
Ph: 1-800-888-8458 / 1-651-681-7600
Fax: 1-651-681-7717
Website: www.ergotron.com

Index

Acid-alkaline balance, 25–30
  monitoring, 30
Acidity, 27–28
  foods for, 27
Acne, 216–217
Acupuncture, 63–64
Aerobic exercise, 21–22
Agency for Toxic Substances and
    Disease Registry, 93
Air, 55–60
  quality, 56–57
  quantity, 56–57
Air bags, 185–186
Air-filtration systems, 59–60
AIDS, 177
ALA. *See* Alpha lipoic acid.
Al-Anon, 84
Alcohol, 11–13, 27, 81–84
  abuse consequences, 83–84
  abuse identification checklist, 83
Alcoholics Anonymous, 84
Alfalfa, 33
Alkalinity, 25–26
  foods for, 26
Alkalize or Die, 28
Allen, James, 208
Allergies, 56–57, 60
Aloe vera, 35
Alpha lipoic acid, 44

Alternative medicine, 61–79
*Alternative Medicine Definitive
    Guide to Cancer,* 139
*Alternative Medicine Definitive
    Guide to Headaches,* 117
Aluminum, 89
American Academy of Pediatrics, 87
American Academy of Sleep
    Medicine, 54
American Cancer Society, 86
American Chiropractic Association,
    67
American Dental Association, 92
American Heart Association, 86, 119
American Holistic Dental
    Association, 68
American Holistic Medical
    Association, 74, 79
American Holistic Nurse's
    Association, 74, 79
American Hospital Association, 78
American Lung Association, 59
American Medical Association:
    Science Reporters Conference,
    86
Anderson, Robert and Jean, 20
Anger, letting go of, 210–211, 219
Animals, 192
Ankylosing spondylitis (AS), 127

Annals of the Rheumatic Diseases,
   126
Anorexia, 123–124
Anthropometrics, 201
Antibiotics, 7–8, 155–156, 159
Antibodies, 158
Antioxidants, 44
Appetite suppressants, 123
Apple Cider Vinegar—Miracle
   Health System, 32
Archives of Pediatrics and
   Adolescent Medicine, 14
Aromatherapy, 64
Arsenic, 92
Arthritis, 125–132
   managing, 131–132
   natural remedies, 129–131
   orthodox treatments, 128
   stress and, 131
   types, 125–128
Arthritis Foundation, 129
Arthritis Trust of America, 130
As a Man Thinketh, 208
Asbestosis, 57
Asbestos, 93
Ascorbic acid. *See* Vitamin C.
Aspartame, 92
Asthma, 145–147
   alternative treatments, 146–147
   conventional treatments,
   145–146
Attitude, 23, 207–220
Automotive safety, 185–187
Ayurvedic medicine, 65

Back in Step: The Road to Recovery
   from Back Pain, 22
Bacterial infections, 159–160
   antibiotics and, 159
probiotics and, 159

Barley grass, 33
Barnes, John, 130
Baroody, Theodore, 28
Barry, Wendell, 168
Baths versus showers, 12
Batmanghelidj, Fereydoon, 13
Beauty of life, 215
Becker, Robert, 157
Beds and mattresses, 45–47
Bee pollen, 33–34
Beliefs, 207–220
Benzene, 93
Beryllium, 93
Beta glucan, 138
Between Heaven and Earth, 66
Beverages, 3–4
Beyond Antibiotics, 160
BGH, 8
Bienfeld and Kornbloom, 66
Blakiston's New Gould Medical
   Dictionary, 161
Blankets, electric, 47
Blaylock, Russell, 92
Blood glucose. *See* Blood sugar.
Blood pressure, 107
Blood pressure test for adrenal
   function, 107
Blood sugar disorders, 103–110
Blueprint for Immortality, 157
Blueprints for Safety, 22
Body, loving your, 216
Body Electric, 157
Body frequencies, 158
Bohr, Niels, 157
Bone marrow transplants, 136
Bonner, Michael, 68
Bootman, J. Lyle, 86
Boswellia, 129
Bovine growth hormone.
   See BGH.

Bradley, Barry, 6
Bragg, Paul and Patricia, 32
Breads, 27
Breathing, 55–60
    deep, 55–56
    posture and, 56
Breggin, Peter R., 71–72
Breiner, Mark, 68
Bromelain, 129
Brown, H. Jackson, 221–222
Brownell, Kelly, 123
Bulimia, 123–124
Burr, Harold Saxon, 157

Cadmium, 91
Caffeine, 11–14, 27
Calcium, 38–40
Calcium citrate, 39
Cancer, 133–139
    alternative medicine for,
        137–139
    diagnosis, 135–136
    early signs, 135
    emotional factors in, 137
    risk factors, 134–135
    Western medicine treatments, 136
Candidiasis, 159
Candy, 27
Carbon monoxide, 188
Carbonated beverages, 27
Cardiopulmonary resuscitation.
    See CPR.
Cardiovascular disease, 95–101
    causes of, 98
Carlson Company, 38
Carnegie, Dale, 215
Carpal tunnel syndrome, 199
Cars, 185–187
    maintenance, 187
Carter-Scot, Cherie, 2

Cave, Stephanie, 88
Cellular starvation, 5–6
Centers for Disease Control, 75,
    86, 88, 121
    National Immunization
        Program, 88
Cereals, 27
Cervicogenic headaches, 115
Chairs, office, 199–200, 204
Change, welcoming, 162
Chelating agent, 89
Chewing, 3–4
Chicken, free-range, 10
Children, 87–88, 174–176
    abuse of, 175–176
    obesity in, 120–122
    parental abuse of, 176
    protecting, 175–176
    raising, 174–175
Chinese medicine. See TCM.
Chiropractic, 17, 66–67, 77
Chiropractic Profession, 67
Chlorella, 34
Chlorine, 15
Chondroitin sulfate, 129
Chopra, Deepak, 65, 157
Cigarette smoke. See Tobacco.
Clark, Hulda, 139
Cleaning solutions, 92–93
Cluster headaches, 114
Coenyzme Q$_{10}$, 44
Coffee, decaf, 14
Colds, 155–160
    prevention, 156
Columbia University Center for
    the Advancement of Children's
    Mental Health, 154
Common sense, 185–198
Commonweal Institute for the
    Study of Health and Illness, 138

Comparing yourself to others, 214–215

Complementary healing, 62–79

Complete Life's Little Instruction Book, 221

Comprehensive Loss Management, Inc., 22

Computer ergonomics, 201–204

Constipation, 141–144
  atonic, 141–143
  consequences of, 144
  irritable bowel syndrome, 141, 143
  stress and, 143–144

Contemporary Chiropractic, 67

Cookbooks, 5

Copy holders, 203

Corn syrup, 27

Cosmetics, 27, 93

Cowden, W. Lee, 139

CPR, 194–195

Cranberries, 27

C-reactive protein. *See* CRP.

Credit card companies, 198

CRP, 97–98

Curcumin, 44, 129

Cure for All Advanced Cancers, 139

Cure for All Cancers, 139

Custards, 27

Dairy products, 10, 27, 39

DDT, 93

DeBecker, Gavin, 176

Dehydration, 11

Dentistry (holistic), 68

Depression, 149–154
  alternative considerations, 150
  recommendations for recovery from, 153
  resources, 154

symptoms, 150
  teenage, 152–154
  work as therapy for, 151

Depression and Bipolar Support Alliance, 154

Devil's claw, 129

Diabetes type I, 103, 122, 123
  children and, 103
  symptoms, 103

Diabetes, type II, 103–105, 123
  children and, 105
  symptoms, 104

Diamond, W. John, 139

Diet, 3–10, 204. *See also* Food.
  stress and, 162
  vegetarian, 9
  weight and, 119–124

Digestion, 3–4

Discovering Homeopathy: Medicine for the 21st Century, 70

Diuretics, 11

Doctors
  selecting, 61–79
  when to visit, 190–191

Donkin, Scott, 205

Dossey, Larry, 101, 208

Dr. Dean Ornish's Program for Reversing Heart Disease, 100

Dreams, 50–54
  interpreting, 51–54

Dreams, Your Magic Mirror, 54

Drugs, 27, 86–88, 192–194. *See also* Over-the-counter drugs.

Drummond, Henry, 173

Eating Disorders and Obesity: A Comprehensive Handbook, 123

EAV, 73

EDS, 60, 72–73, 147, 154

Education, furthering, 164

EFAs, 97, 154
Eggs, 10, 27
Einstein, Albert, 157
Eisenberg, David, 76
Electrical hazards, 187–188
Electrical Nutrition, 160
Electro-acupuncture by Voll. *See* EAV.
Electro-dermal screening. *See* EDS.
Eli Lilly and Company, 90
Emerson, Ralph Waldo, 222
Emphysema, 57
Endocrine system, 109–110
Energy, 201–202
Enkephalins, 152
EnTerra, 43
Environmental Protection Agency. *See* U.S. Environmental Protection Agency.
Environne Fruit and Vegetable Wash, 7
Enzyme Nutrition, 44
Enzymes, 43
Epstein, Samuel, 138
Equipment, protective, 187
Erasmus, Udo, 32
Ergonomics, 199–205
    overview, 205
Ergotron, 205
Essential fatty acids. *See* EFAs.
Estrogen, 40–41
ETA, 129
Ewing, Dawn, 68
Exercise, 17–23
Exotoxins: The Taste That Kills, 92
Eye exercises, 203
Eye strain, preventing, 202–203
Eye glasses, 203

Fairburn, Chris, 123

Faith, 211–212
Falls, trips and slips, 196–197
Fast food, 120–121
Fast Food Nation, 121
Father Sebastian Kneipp Health Spa, 70
Fats, 96–97
    polyunsaturated, 96
    saturated, 96
Fats That Heal, Fats That Kill, 32
Fetal alcohol syndrome, 82
Field, The, 157
Fillings, amalgam, 68
Fink, John, 138
Finland, 122
Fire hazards, 187–188
Firearms, 195
First, Do No Harm, 74–75
Fish, 10, 27
Flaxseeds, 44
Flour, white, 27
Flouride, 15, 91–92
Flouride Action Network, 92
Flu, 155–160
    prevention, 156
Folate. *See* Folic acid.
Folic acid, 5,
Fontana, David, 54
Food Enzymes for Health and Longevity, 44
Food, 3–10, 31–36, 96–97. *See also* Diet.
    genetically engineered, 7–9
    irradiated, 7
    organic, 6–7, 9
    selection, 6
Forgiveness, 210
Formaldehyde, 93
Fox, J. Emmet, 173
Frequencies, body, 158

Freud, Sigmund, 72
Friendship, 178–184
    checklist for good, 179–181
    checklist for bad, 182–184
Fruits, 7, 9, 26, 27
    juices, 13–14, 26
    peeling, 7
Fungicide, 7
Future, choosing, 210

Garlic, 31–32
Genetically engineered foods, 7–9
Gerber, Richard, 157
Germs, 156–159
Gibran, Kahil, 165, 207
Ginger root extract, 129
Ginkgo biloba, 35
Ginseng, 35
Glucosamine sulfate, 129
Glucose. See Blood sugar.
Goldberg, Burton, 117, 139
Gouty arthritis, 127–128
Grace, 184
Grains, 27
Grasses, 33
Graston technique, 130
Gratitude, 210
Greatest Thing in the World, 173
Grocery store lists, 10
Gum chewing, 4

Hahnemann, Samuel, 68
Hair dyes, 126–127
Hale, Lindsey, 124
Harmony in relationships, 169–170
Harvard University, 14, 40, 41
    Medical School, 76
    School of Public Health, 36
Hawkins, David R., 72
Headaches, 111–117

natural approaches to treating,
    117
nutrients for prevention, 116
types, 111–115
Healing Words, the Power of
    Prayer and the Practice of
    Medicine, 208
Healthcare alternatives, 61–79
Healthy Living Space, 60
Heart attacks, 98–99
Heart disease, 95–101
    causes, 98
Heart pulse, 21
Heat for arthritis, 131
Heat versus ice to reduce
    headaches, 115–116
Heat exhaustion, 189–190
Heatstroke, 189–190
Heavy metals. See Metals, heavy.
Heimlich maneuver, 194–195
Heisenberg, Werner, 157
Helmets, 186
Herbicides, 7
Hiestand, Denie and Shelley, 160
Hippocrates, 10, 36, 69, 70
Hobbies and stress, 163
Holistic Dental Association, 68
Holistic health care, 61–62
Holmes, Thomas, 170–171
Holmes-Rahe Social Readjustment
    Rating Scale, 171
Holmes-Rahe stress inventory,
    170–171
Homeopathy, 68
Homocysteine, 97
Homocysteine Revolution, 97
Honey, raw non-pateurized, 33
Hormone replacement therapy,
    40–41
Hormones, 7, 40–41

Horton's Syndrome, 114
Household cleaners and solvents, 92–93
How to Be Your Own Doctor—Sometimes, 62
How to Raise a Healthy Child in Spite of Your Doctor, 88
How to Stop Worrying and Start Living, 215
Howell, Edward, 44
Huang Ti Nei-Ching, 65
Huggins, Hal, 68
Human nature, 167
Hurrying through life, 212
Hydration, 11,
Hypoglycemia, 105–109, 154
    clinical management of, 107–109
    diagnosing, 106–107
    foods for, 108–109
    foods to avoid, 109
    functional testing for, 106
    laboratory testing for, 106

Ice versus heat to reduce headaches, 115–116
Idiopathic polyneuropathy, 87
If Life Is a Game, These Are the Rules, 2
Illness and positive attitude, 214
Immune system, 137, 158–159
Immunizations, 87
Immunizations: The Terrible Risks Your Children Face That Your Doctor Won't Reveal, 88
Infections, 155–160
    natural approaches to, 160
Innate intelligence, 66
Insomnia, 48
Inspired to Lose, 123
Institute of Medicine, 82

Insulin, 104–105
Insulin regulation, 104–105
International Academy of Chiropractic Occupational Health Consultants, 131, 205
Irish Cancer Society, 86
Irradiated foods, 7
Irritable bowel syndrome (IBS), 143
It's All in Your Head, 68

Jacob Wetterling Foundation, 176
Jenner, Edward, 69
Joint health, 12
Journal of the American Medical Association, 41, 86
Jung, Carl, 72
Junk food, 120–121
Juvenile arthritis, 127

Kaiser Permanente, 75
Kapchuk, Ted, 66
Ketchup, 27
Key-E Kaps, 38
KWAI garlic, 32
Kyolic garlic, 32

Lamb, 10
Laughing, 164–165
Lawrence, David, 75
Lead, 90–91, 151
    and children, 90
Lead paint, 90
Lead pipes, 91
Lee, John, 41
Legionnaire's disease, 57
Legumes, 27
Let the Tooth Be Known, 68
Leviton, Richard, 60
Life, beauty of, 215

Life Source Basics, 138
Lifestyle, 95–96, 162–170, 173–184,
    204, 207–220
Light reflex pupil response test,
    106–107
Lighting, 202
Lightning, 197
Lincoln, Abraham, 151–152
Lipoic acid. *See* Alpha lipoic acid.
Living abundantly, 213
Living in the moment, 168–169
Living your dreams, 213
Los Angeles Times, 75
Lundberg, Gary and Joy, 174
Lust, Benedict, 70

Mad Farmer, 169
Magnesium, 40, 41–42, 154
Margarine, 27
Marriage, 174
Married for Better, Not Worse—
    The Fourteen Secrets to a
    Happy Marriage, 174
Massage, 18
    deep-tissue, 19
Mayonnaise, 27
McCully, Kilmer, 97
McTaggart, Lynne, 157
MCS, 58
    resources for, 60
Meat, 10, 27
Medicine cabinet inventories, 192
Meditation, 168
Melnik, Michael, 22
Mendelsohn, Robert, 88
Menopause, 40–41
Mercury, 89–90
Meridians, 63
Metals, heavy, 88–92
Methyl chloride, 93

Methyl sulfylmethane (MSM), 129
Meyer, Gérard, 205
Microwave ovens, 197
Migraine headache, 112
    recommendations to reduce,
        112
Milk, 13. *See also* Dairy products.
Milne, Robert, 117
Minerals, 37–44
Mitchell, Deborah, 88
Molecules of Emotion, 158
Monosodium glutamate (MSG), 92
More, Blake, 117
Multiple chemical sensitivity. *See*
    MCS.
Murphy, Jamie, 88
Muscle stripping, 18–19
Myofascial release therapy, 130

Narcotics Anonymous, 84
National Academy of Sciences,
    Institute of Medicine, 82
National Association of Anorexia
    Nervosa and Associated
    Disorders, 124
National Cancer Institute, 135,
    136
National Center for Missing and
    Exploited Children, 176
National Eating Disorders
    Association, 124
National Exchange Club Centers
    for the Prevention of Child
    Abuse, 176
National Highway Traffic
    Administration, 186
National Institute for Occupational
    Safety and Health, 205
National Institute of Mental Health,
    153

National Mental Health Awareness Campaign, 154
National Press Club, 75
National Research Council, 86
National Safety Council, 186
National Stroke Association, 100
National Vaccine Information Center, 88
Natural healing, 61–79
Nature's design, respect for, 5
Naturopathic medicine, 70
Necterra Plus, 28, 43
Neurologists, when to consult for headaches, 116
Neurology, 87
New Balance shoes, 21
Neways International, 93
Nicotine, 85–86
No thank you, 5
Norway, 121
NSAIDs, 87, 128
Nutrition. *See* Diet.
Nutritional consultants, 6
Nutritional supplements. *See* Supplements.
Nuts, 26, 27

Oat grass, 33
Obesity, 5–123
in children, 120–121
Occupational Safety & Health Administration. *See* OSHA.
Office chairs, 199–200, 204
Office computers, 201–205
Office desks, 200–201
Office ergonomics, 199–205
Oils, 26, 96–97
hydrogenated, 27, 96–97
Onions, 32
Opening Your Heart, 101

Oral Health Bible, 68
Organic food, 6–7
Ornish, Dean, 100–101
Orthomolecular psychiatry, 72
OSHA, 22, 199
Oslay, Ted, 130
Osteoarthritis, 125–126
Osteopathy, 17, 70–71
cranial, 71
craniosacral therapy, 71
Osteoporosis, 40–41
Ostroff, Martha, 124
Overcoming Binge Eating, 123
Overeaters Anonymous, 123
Over-the-counter drugs, 87, 128, 192–194. *See also* Drugs.
Overweight, 5
Ownership, reconsidering, 215
Oxygen, 55–56
Ozone generators, 59–60

Pain, attitude toward, 194
Palmer, David Daniel, 66
Paraquat, 93
Pastas, 27
Pasteur, Louis, 159
Patient's Bill of Rights, 77–78
Pauling, Linus, 72
Peak Performance Body & Mind, 205
Pediatrics, 87–88
Perfect Health—The Complete Mind/Body Guide, 65
Personal care products, 92–93
Pert, Candace, 158
Pesticides, 7
pH, 25–30
pH balance. *See* Acid-alkaline balance.
Phytonadione. *See* Vitamin K.

Pillows, 47

Plasma₂ Monitor and Keyboard
    Positioning Unit, 204

Play, 166–167

Pleasure, 213

Poison Control Center, 90

Poison control chart, 192–193

Poisons in body, 81–93

Politics of Cancer Revisited, 138

Posner, Trisha, 41

Posture, 202

    breathing and, 56

Potassium, 42

Potentization, 69

Power foods. *See* Foods.

Power of Now, 169, 170

*Practical Guide to Vibrational
    Medicine,* 157

Practice of Aromatherapy, 64

Prayer, 207–208

Pregnancy, 82

Prescription drugs. *See* Drugs.

Probiotics, 159

Progesterone, 40–41

Property protection, 197–198

Prophet, The, 165

Protecting the Gift, 176

Protective equipment, 187

Proteins, 9–10

    non-vegetable sources, 10

Prozac, 151

Prudence, 212

Psoriatric arthritis, 128

Psychiatry, 71–72

Psychotherapy, 72

Qigong, 73

Quantum Healing, 157

Quicksilver. *See* Mercury.

Quotes, 221–222

Radon, 93

Rahe, Richard, 171

Rankin, Howard, 123

Rebound headaches, 115

Redwood, Daniel, 67

Refrigerator, cleaning out, 195–196

Reiki, 73

Relationship harmony, 169–170

Relationships, 173–184

Relaxation techniques, 76

Religion, 211–212

REM sleep, 49–50

Remen, Rachel Naomi, 138

Resistance to life and stress, 163

Respiration, 21, 55–60

    diseases, 56–59, 145–147

Respondex, 130–131

Rest, 45–54

Resveratrol, 44

Retreats, 212–213

Rheumatoid arthritis, adult, 126

Risk-taking, 167

Rogers, Will, 167

Rolfing, 74

Romm, Aviva Jill, 88

Room lighting, 202

Royal jelly, 34

Running, 20

Rye grass, 33

S-adenosyl methionine (SAM-e),
    129, 151

Sadness, 164

Saliva, 3–4, 30

SAM-e. *See* S-adenosyl methionine
    (SAM-e).

Schlosser, Eric, 121

Schmidt, Michael, 154, 160

Schrodinger, Erwin, 157

Sciatica, 196

Screen glare, reducing, 202
Seafood, 10, 27
Seasonal affective disorder (SAD), 152
Seasoning, 26
Seat belts, 185–186
Sechrist, Elsie, 54
Secondhand smoke, 85–86
Secret Language of Dreams, 54
Sehnert, Keith, 62
Selenium, 44
Self-esteem, 122–123, 213–214
Septic or infectious arthritis, 128
Serotonin, 123
Sex, 177
    abuse, 177
Sexually transmitted diseases (STDs), 177
Shames, Karilee Halo, 110
Shames, Richard L., 110
Shealy, Norman, 74
Shock, 190
Shoes, 20–21
Sick-building syndrome, 57–58
Silicosis, 57
Silver Dental Fillings—The Toxic Time Bomb, 68
Sinus headaches, 114
Sitting on the Job, 205
Sleep, 45–54
    deep, 50
    dreams and, 50–54
    postures, 47
    problems, 48–49
    REM, 49
Slips, trips, and falls, 195–197
Smart Fats, 154
Smith, David Chapman, 67
Smoking. *See* Tobacco.
Smoothie recipes, 29

Sodas, 14
Sodium chloride, 42
Soft drinks, 14
Solvents, 92–93
Somatoform disorder, 219
Soy lecithin, 34
Spastic constipation. *See* Irritable bowel syndrome.
Spina bifida, 5
Spine health, 12, 17–18
Spine injuries, preventing, 22
Spirulina, 34
St. John's wort, 151
Stance Angle Chair and Plasma$_2$ Monitor and Keyboard Positioning Unit, 204
Standard American diet, 122
Statin drugs, 87
Stem cells, 136
Still, Andrew Taylor, 70
Stress, 131, 143, 147, 161–171
    diet and, 162
    Holmes-Rahe inventory, 170–171
    overcoming, 162–170
    work and, 165–166
Stretching, 19–20
Stretching, 20
Stroke, 99–100
    warning signs, 99–100
Subluxation complex, 67
Sugar, 13–14, 26, 27, 27. *See also* Blood sugar.
Suicide, 152, 154
Sunlight, 152, 188–189
Sunstroke, 189–190
Supplements, 37–44, 97, 123
    buying and using, 43
    time-release, 43
Sutherland, William, 71

Sweden, 121

Sweeteners, 14, 26, 27, 92

Swimming, 131

Systemic disease, 137

Take Off Pounds Sensibly (TOPS), 123

TCM, 63–64, 65, 155

Tea
 black, 27
 herbal, 13, 26

Teenagers, 152–154, 186

10 Hidden Reasons You Are Sick— And What to Do About Them, 6

Temporomadibular joint. See TMJ.

Tension headaches, 111–112

Therapy Care Resources, 130

Third Opinion, 138

This Is Not Your Mother's Menopause, 41

Thoreau, Henry David, 167

Thoughts, 207–208

Thunderstorms, 197

Thymus gland, 109–110

Thyroid hormone replacement, 109–110

Thyroid Power—10 Steps to Total Health, 110

Time management, 163, 212

TMJ, 4, 113–114
 headaches and, 113

Tobacco, 27, 57, 85–86, 96

Tolle, Eckhart, 169, 170

Toxic Psychiatry, 71

Toxins, 81–93

Traditional Chinese medicine. See TCM.

Transcendental meditation, 168

Trips, slips and falls, 196

Turkey, free-range, 10

Udo's Choice Perfected Oil Blend, 32, 97

Ullman, Dana, 70

Undernourishment, 5–7

United Way's First Call for Help, 84

University of Arizona College of Pharmacy, 86

University of Washington, 170

Upledger, John, 71

U.S. Army, 165

U.S. Bureau of Labor Statistics, 199

U.S. Department of Agriculture, 6, 10

U.S. Environmental Protection Agency, 91

U.S. Food and Drug Administration, 60, 86, 91, 92, 193

U.S. Surgeon General, 120–121

Vaccinations, 87

Vaccinations, 88

Valnet, 64

Vegetables, 7, 9, 26
 juices, 13–14, 26

Vegetarian diet, 9

Vehicular safety, 185–187

Vibrational medicine, 157

Vibrations, body, 158

Vinegar
 cider, 32–33
 white, 27

Viruses, 155–159

Visualization, 208–210

Vitamin A, 37, 44

Vitamin C, 38, 40, 44, 89

Vitamin D, 37, 40, 122, 188

Vitamin E, 37–38, 44

Vitamin K, 37

Vitamins, 37–44
 multi, with minerals, 43
 time-release, 43

Voll, Reinhold, 73
Voll testing, 72–73

Walking, 20
Washing produce, 7
Water, 11–16
  aging and, 13
  bottled, 15
  distilled, 14–15
  filtered, 16
  flouridated, 91–92
  joint health and, 12–13
  municipal tap, 15
  nerves and, 13
  reverse-osmosis, 14–15
  well, 15
Water substitutes, 13–14
Weapons, 195
Web That Has No Weaver, 66
Weight, 119–124
Weight-loss books, 5
Weight-loss programs, 120
Weight training, 22
What Every Parent Should Know About Childhood Immunization, 88
What Your Doctor May Not Tell You About Children's Vaccinations, 88
What Your Doctor May Not Tell You About Menopause, 41

What Your Doctor May Not Tell You About Pre-Menopause, 41
Wheat, 27
Wheat grass, 33
Whining, 212
White, Carol, 88
White willow bark extract, 129
Whole Body Dentistry, 68
Women's Health Initiative, 41
Wonder foods, 31–36
Work
  and ergonomics, 199–205
  and stress, 165–166
  as therapy, 151
  breaks, 203–204
  posture, 202
Work-related injuries, 196–197
Workstations, 199–205
World Health Organization, 1, 86
Wrinkles, 13

Yellow Emperor's Manual of Internal Medicine, 65
Yoga, 167–168
Your Body's Many Cries for Water, 13
Youth Depression Screening Initiative, 154

Ziff, Sam, 68
Zoloft, 151

About the Author

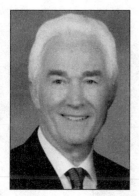

Joseph J. Sweere, D.C., is a graduate of Northwestern Health Sciences University in Bloomington, Minnesota, where he is a full-time professor in the Clinical Sciences Division and chairman of the Department of Occupational Health. He is a diplomate of both the American Board of Chiropractic Orthopedists and the American Chiropractic Board of Occupational Health, and is a fellow of the International College of Chiropractic.

His many memberships include the American Public Health Association, and in 1994, he was named to the Advisory Council of the International Federation for Holistic Health. The recipient of numerous awards and honors, Dr. Sweere served as editor of *Chiropractic Family Practice—A Clinical Manual,* and has authored dozens of papers and articles for professional publications. He has lectured at health forums and conferences in forty-three states, Australia, Canada, Cuba, England, Mexico, Norway, and Switzerland. He has also participated in numerous radio, newspaper, and television interviews, and has been quoted on health-related topics in *The New York Times, The Wall Street Journal, The Minneapolis Star and Tribune,* and the *Reader's Digest.*

Dr. Sweere has more than forty years of experience as a healthcare provider, author, and lecturer, and is considered a leading authority on the art, science, and philosophy of chiropractic, as well as occupational-health education.